G000293133

# INTRODUCTION

While staying in Africa during 1973/4 I came into contact with a lady who was very interested in alternative therapies. Knowing my background in the Health and Beauty profession she lent me a book to read "Stories The Feet Can Tell", which had been written in 1938 by the famous American Reflexologist Eunice Ingham.

I was particularly fascinated by the book because as a child in Ireland, where folk medicine and folk-lore were part of life, I had met so many people who had the cure for so many ills. There were cures for "warts, the pains and chilblains" to name but a few and the bone setter was always on hand for the slipped disc or broken leg whether it be man or beast that was affected.

In my own case I had been told to massage my feet for chilblains and wear sheep's wool in my shoes.

For headaches we massaged our thumbs or around the base of the head (The Occipital) or around the eyes.

For worries such as school exams my late mother told me to massage my hands and wring them out. I still find myself following that same routine of hand massage more than thirty five years later. I realised on reading the Eunice Ingham Book that my hand massage of childhood bore a remarkable resemblance to the massage being described in Eunice Ingham's book.

On pointing out my interest to Edie who had given me the book, she invited me to learn the subject "first hand." Her knowledge had been gained from years of interest in the subject of health both through the natives of Africa and an American medical couple she had met in Zambia in the early sixties. I worked with and learned from Edie during the year that followed. When I left Africa in the summer of 1974 Edie gave me her proud possession of documented case studies. I placed them together with the many studies I had now collected for myself in an old brown attaché case to carry back with me to England rather than entrust them to transport with the risk of getting lost.

On the overland journey home to England while I ate my supper in a small outback hotel in the Province of Natal my car window was broken and the brown attaché case which had been carefully hidden under some blankets in the rear of our family estate was stolen, together with the blankets I had used to disguise them.

To my husband's delight however, all the camera equipment, which also lay beneath the blankets remained intact and untouched.

On my return to England my interest in the subject grew, as did my expansion of friends, though some were very sceptical at first.

In 1975 when Doreen Bailey gave me two treatments for sciatica, a condition that reared its ugly head after the birth of my second son in 1967, the results of the treatment served only to strengthen my belief and determination to succeed in spreading the knowledge and treatment.

Doreen and I spent some time on each of my two visits (2 complete days) discussing the treatment, its benefits and limitations; as well as ways in which we might educate the British public into recognizing the values of this ancient therapy.

During my eighteen years gaining experience in Reflexology and having treated some thousands of people and personally trained numerous therapists (in latter years to pass the examinations of the International Examinations Board, I.E.B. and for membership of the International Federation of Reflexologists, I.F.R.), I have been aware that there is still a need for a simple to follow guide on a no nonsense routine which will also help to dispel some of the mystery which surrounds this treatment.

Reflexology is a treatment that can be performed by most people; especially those who are prepared to study a basic course in anatomy and physiology and use their commonsense with regard to orthodox medicine.

This book will be of help to the the lay person who wishes to treat family and friends and also an asset to the Student or Qualified Therapist who wishes to work as a Professional.

# A BRIEF HISTORY OF REFLEXOLOGY

The true origins of this treatment or folk medicine are unknown but like some of the other complementary therapies it is gradually becoming respectable.

It is believed to be almost as old as history itself. We know this treatment was practised in India and China more than three thousand years ago (3000).

In Egypt a wall painting was found in the Tomb of the Physicians dating back to 2330BC. The painting depicts Reflexology or foot and hand pressure massage.

This form of pressure therapy is still used by the Indian tribes in the way it was practised by their forefathers centuries ago.

The great Florentine Sculptor Cellini who lived between 1500 and 1571 used pressure on hands and feet to relieve pain; as did the 20th American President W. Garfield (1831-1881).

The ancient therapy was established in America more or less in its present form by the American Physician Dr. William Fitzgerald (1872-1942).

In 1917 Dr Fitzgerald and Dr. Edwin Bowers published a book called "Zone Therapy, relieving pain at home".

Dr Fitzgerald gave courses and seminars on his work and many Americans became both followers and believers of this ancient Therapy. It was practised by members of the medical profession and lay people alike.

A young lady Masseuse named Eunice Ingham became interested in the Ancient Therapy. Encouraged and taught by her friends and employers Dr. Riley and his wife, she took the work very seriously and was unstinting with time and effort in collecting data and information from her own and colleagues' experiences.

Eunice developed a pressure massage which she called "The Ingham Method". She published two books. Her first in 1938 "Stories the Feet can Tell" and in 1963 "Stories the Feet have Told". Sadly in 1974 Eunice Ingham died.

Doreen Bailey, a former student of Eunice Ingham returned to England from America in 1966 and became the pioneer of Reflexology in this country.

In 1975 I had the pleasure of meeting Doreen and from that day forwards I was determined to study, practise and teach this Ancient Natural Therapy.

In this book I, like my predecessors, make changes to the routine and treatment and, like them, the changes are based on experience.

# REFLEXOLOGY EXPLAINED

Reflexology is the technique of pressure massage to the feet or hands where all the internal body structures and organs are mirrored. It is a simple non-invasive treatment which helps the body to maintain a delicate balance between the nine systems.

1 Skeletal
2 Muscular
3 Vascular
4 Neurological
5 Respiratory
6 Digestive
7 Endocrine
8 Genito
9 Reproductive

All these systems work together in harmony and unison to keep us in a state of good health.

No one knows exactly how Reflexology works, although many theories exist. Most Reflexologists subscribe to the theory that the body is divided into ten longitudinal zones (or energy channels). These zones are lines running the entire length of the body; five on each side of the median line (an imaginary line running from the crown of the head to between the feet-see diagram 'A'-page 10).

These zones extent into the feet which are also divided into ten zones five on each foot. (see diagram 'D' - page 12). The foot zones are located with number one on the first toe (big toe) counting to number five on the little toe. These lines are repeated, running down the arm to the fingers. (see diagram 'C' - page 19). On the hands number one zone or channel runs to the thumb and number five to the little finger.

Energy is constantly flowing through these zones or channels. On each foot and hand are found reflex points that correspond to each gland and structure in the body.

The hands and feet have the same reflex zones and points, however from working experience there is no doubt that treatment of the feet gives better therapeutic results than does treatment of the hands. While all therapists believe in the benefits of the treatment there are some who believe that because of the mobility of the hand the reflexes are not so clearly defined. Yet another school of thought is that because the total body weight passes through the feet the energy channels or reflex points are more sensitive.

The reflex points of Reflexology differ from the reflex points of the nervous system. They do not cross the spinal column and are invisible on dissection and to X-ray.

It could therefore be said that in this instance reflex is taken to mean the reflection of the organs of the body in miniature on the feet.

When the energy flow is blocked by congestion, disorders and even disease can occur. Crystalline deposits will sometimes form on the corresponding reflex point on the hand and the foot. When the therapists treats a reflex point, one aim is to break down these crystals; the energy flow is thus enhanced, encouraging the systems to work again in unison.

Besides the ten energy channels already mentioned three further lines should be taken into consideration. These are the imaginary lateral lines that traverse the foot (or hand). ( See diagram 'B' - page 11 ). These lines help the reflexologist to make a map of the foot or indeed the body. It is worth bearing in mind that the shape and size of feet differ in each individual. Therefore if treatment is always started by first visualising these three imaginary lines on the feet then it is easy to work out the reflexes that are above or below these lines.

| | |
|---|---|
| 1 The diaphragm line | Just below the ball of the foot. |
| 2 The waist line. | In the centre of the arch. |
| 3 The pelvic floor line. | On the heel where thickness of the flesh changes to softness. |

All organs and structures above the diaphragm on the body will have their reflex point above the diaphragm line on the foot and all organs below the diaphragm will have the reflex point in the corresponding area on the foot.

These three horizontal or transverse lines could logically be placed almost anywhere on the foot by a therapist with a very good working knowledge of anatomy and physiology. However the most commonly used three lines, which in turn form compartments for the organs of areas of the body, are the ones mentioned and are the ones which I personally use.

The alternative areas commonly used are as follows

1 The shoulder girdle line.

2 The waist line.

3 The pelvic line.

Organs on the right side of the body will be found in the right foot and those on the left side of the body found in the left foot.

Where two organs exists, for example two lungs, then they will be found one on each foot.

Likewise where the organ crosses the midline in the body it will then be found on both feet.

The reflex zone to an organ can be found occupying the same vertical body zone in the feet as the organ occupies in the body.

## THE WORKING THERAPIST

All Reflexologists whether working for family and friends or as professional therapists need to have a basic knowledge of anatomy and physiology. The professional therapist needs to have a very good working knowledge of the body's structures and functions and should make an effort to study this subject to the acceptable standard. Therapists with membership of a professional Reflexology organisation will have undertaken a course of study in anatomy and physiology over and above the study of Reflexology, under a qualified tutor.

7

Furthermore Reflexology organisations such as I.F.R. require that students undertake a considerable number of hours of case study work before embarking on a career as a therapist.

It is true to say that a qualified therapist will not mix his/her therapies in any one  session; to do so would be overstimulating.

Too much stimulation can have a bad effect, but as I have said before Reflexology is not a ' Cure All ' to the exclusion of all other therapies. To insist on it being so indicates a lack of ability to evaluate the relative worth of different possibilities.

I would always advise that if you are treating others in a professional capacity you undertake a full course of training in that subject to a qualifing standard and never offer any treatment or part of any treatment beyond that in which you hold a qualification.

# SOME BENEFITS OF REFLEXOLOGY

Calms and Soothes

Gives the client a feeling of wellbeing

Improves circulation

Relaxes mind and body

Removes waste deposits that have built up on the reflex points

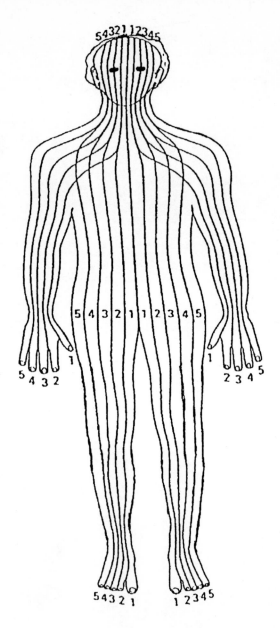

**DIAGRAM A**

# TRANSVERSE LINES

## RIGHT FOOT                         LEFT FOOT

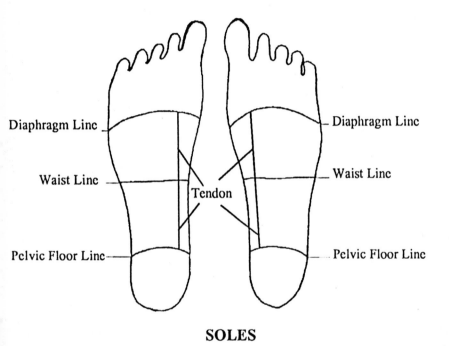

**SOLES**

**DIAGRAM 'B'**

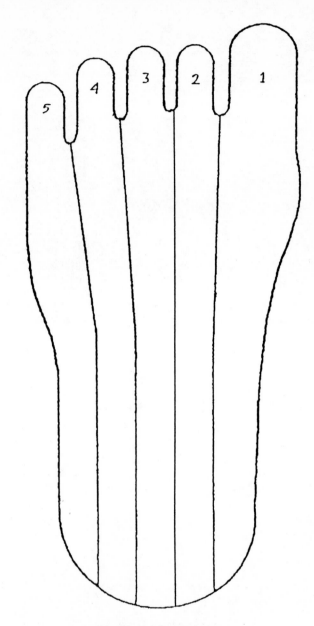

**ZONES OF THE FOOT**

**DIAGRAM 'D'**

MIRROR OF THE BODY

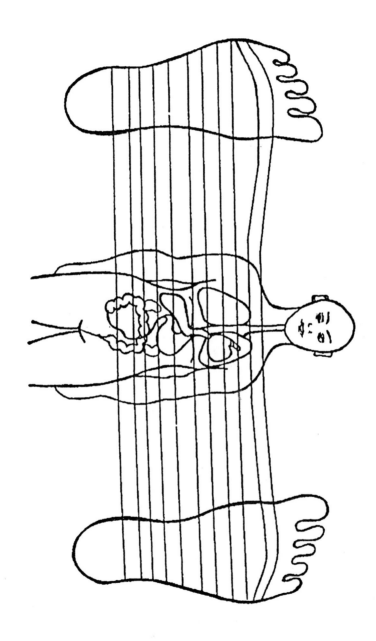

# THE STRUCTURE OF THE FOOT

| | | | |
|---|---|---|---|
| 7 | TARSALS | **NOTE.** | |
| 5 | METATARSALS | | ONLY 2 PHALANGES IN |
| 14 | PHALANGES | | THE BIG TOE |

Besides these 26 bones the foot also contains
21    MUSCLES
50    LIGAMENTS
500    BLOOD VESSELS
500    NERVES

The bones of the foot are so arranged as to produce three distinct arches :

**THE MEDIAL** Longitudinal Arch.
This is the highest of the arches and is formed by the :
TALUS
CALCANEUS
NAVICULAR
Three CUNIFORM BONES and METATARSALS numbers 1,2,3.
Only the Calcaneus and the distal end of the Metatarsal should touch the ground.

**THE LATERAL** Longitudal Arch
This is much less marked than the Medial Arch and is composed of the :
CALCANEUS
CUBOID and
METATARSALS 4,5.

**THE TRAVERSE** Arch
This arch is formed by the :
NAVICULAR
Three CUNIFORM
CUBOID
METATARSALS 1 to 5

The Arches are not fixed, they give as the weight of the body is transmitted to the ground. When the weight is removed they return to their original state.

The bones comprising the arches are held in position by ligaments and tendons. When these ligaments and tendons are weakened the height of the Medial Longitudinal Arch may decrease or 'fall' causing Flat Foot.

# THE STRUCTURE OF THE FOOT

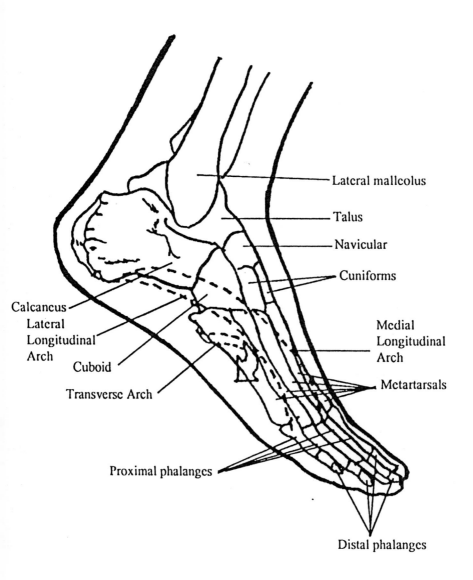

Lateral malleolus

Talus

Navicular

Cuniforms

Calcaneus

Lateral
Longitudinal
Arch

Medial
Longitudinal
Arch

Cuboid

Metartarsals

Transverse Arch

Proximal phalanges

Distal phalanges

**WEIGHT BEARING
BONES OF THE FOOT
OUTLINED BY
TRIANGLE**

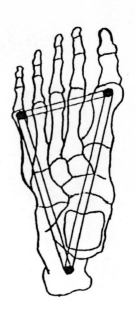

**CUSHIONED WEIGHT
BEARING AREA OF THE
FOOT**

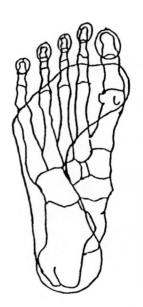

# REFERRAL
# ZONES

# REFERRAL ZONES

Referral zones are an important part of treatment, particularly when treating oneself or dealing with cases of injury or infection; when the normal area cannot be treated.

For Example

Fingers Treat Toes

Hands Treat Foot

Wrist Treat Ankle

Forearm Treat Calf

Elbow Treat Knee

Upper Arm Treat Thigh

Shoulder Treat Hip

Naturally these treatments can be performed in reverse order. In the case of a Knee injury one could treat the Elbow; and so on.

When you know the Longitudinal Zones then the next step is to trace the zone in which that part of the body lies that is causing the problem. A general massage of the Referral Zone should bring relief to the area of the body that is out of tune. (see diagram 'C' - page19).

It is worth bearing in mind that self-treatment, while being helpful, will never be as beneficial as a treatment given by another; as it is impossible to achieve the same degree of relaxation and equally as difficult to perceive one's own bodily reactions.

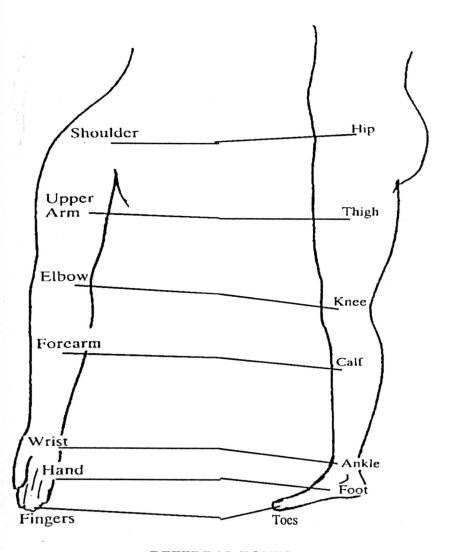

**REFERRAL ZONES**

**DIAGRAM 'C '**

# WHAT ARE THE CRYSTALS?

Uric Acid and excess Calcium are two of the waste products that build up in the body when the metabolism is not working according to plan. These deposits can be felt on the feet as grains of sugar or sand. The little clumps can be broken down by Reflexology Massage. The broken down deposits are then carried by the blood and lymph flow to be eliminated by the body.

# WHEN TREATMENTS MUST NOT BE PERFORMED

This list of contra indications and precautions is meant to be a guide and is in no way to be taken as full and complete. The responsibility for the client rests with the therapist using his/her commonsense at all times.

For any condition currently being treated by a medically qualified person without first obtaining that person's consent.

Immediately prior to or directly after surgery.

Pregnancy. Where there is any element of risk and never without medical consent. All movements should be light.

In cases of infectious or contagious conditions.

Herpies Zooster (Shingles). During active phase.

Undiagnosed pain especially acute.

Thrombosis, Phlebitis.

Directly over an area of varicose veins.

After a heavy meal (within a couple of hours).

On an empty stomach. Offer a glass of fruit juice and a biscuit.

On a person under the influence of the abuse of Alcohol or Drugs.

On a person taking strong medication. (advise client to get medical consent).

During menstruation if it is normally heavy.

For any rare or unusual condition without prior medical consent.

Remember it is not within the skill of a Reflexologist to diagnose. That is the prerogative of the medically qualified or others recognised to do so.

# WHEN TO EXERCISE CAUTION

Epileptics. Client might have a fit. Can you cope?

When working on a diabetic use less pressure than normal and work for only about twenty minutes in total. Care should be taken in the Pancreas area (treated with stomach) as there is a possibility of triggering off Insulin shock if the pressures are too heavy or prolonged.

Do not treat with pressure circles on sensitive points but hold and release once.

Diabetics have a slow healing rate; heavy pressure might cause bruising.

The Diabetic skin is easily broken or torn. Should this happen then the person might get a varicose ulcer.

It is possible to release too many Toxins for the system to cope with and this can make the Diabetic feel ill.

**Under normal circumstances** when the client has a high Crystalline deposit or is very sensitive to touch, to over-treat would cause a similar reaction as to that of the diabetic.

In order to overcome this, it is advisable to treat the client for a shorter period of time, increasing the pressure circles from one or two to begin with to the normal seven as the course progresses.
This should give the body a chance to disperse the Toxins.

Pregnancy has been mentioned as a possible Contra Indication. It can however be a beneficial treatment during labour and immediately after delivery, providing there are no medical complications; the therapist is fully qualified and both patient and medical consent has been granted to allow the treatment to be performed.

All practitioners of Reflexology should be aware not only of its benefits but also of its limitations.

It is of the utmost importance to exercise caution when dealing with the health of others.

Be prepared to refer people to their Doctor or other Practitioners when necessary.

Never diagnose.

Never make false claims for the treatment.

And above all, never give false hope.

**Take extra care when dealing with Children, the Elderly, the Terminally Ill, Diabetic, unusual conditions, acute conditions ( know and do not treat the notifiable diseases without special medical consent).**

# SOME DO'S AND DO NOT'S OF REFLEXOLOGY

## THE DO NOT'S

Work on tendons or bone. ( With heavy pressure )

Work on infected areas.

Work on broken skin.

Work over surface veins.

Work over recent scar tissue.

Increase greatly the depth of pressure when you feel a Crystal.

Hurt client to extent of causing deep pain or discomfort.

Diagnose disorder or a disease.

Tell client the organ that corresponds to the Crystal.

Give false hope.

Make false claims.

Have a flustered, rushed or hurried approach to your work.

Discuss one client with another.

Abuse your professional position.

Set up and work as a professional Reflexologist unless you have the necessary training, hold the qualification of a recognised Examinations Authority, and belong to a professional organisation.

# SOME DO'S AND DO NOT'S OF REFLEXOLOGY

## THE DO'S

Take care of your client.

Give each and every client your undivided attention.

Be honest as far as possible.

Have a warm, clean and relaxed atmosphere to work in.

Have a soothing, calm, quiet voice.

Explain clearly to the client what you would like them to do. For example remove shoes, socks, tights, lie down, bend leg.

Give a helping hand to the less able in removing shoes and clothing.

Try to accommodate clients who might have a strict timetable to adhere to. Parking meters, public transport or dental appointments do not wait.

Complete consultation card prior to treatment and therapy record card on completion of treatment, while client is getting ready to leave, or immediately after their departure.

Respect your client's shyness and confidentiality.

# KNOW YOUR RESPONSIBILITIES

If you take it upon yourself to tell your client the precise organs you are working on, then you should be prepared to take the consequences of your action. ( The International Federation of Reflexologists ( I.F.R.) advise against telling clients the specific organs being worked on )

Many clients who seem calm, logical and sensible while in your company can be caused great anxiety when alone, thinking about your treatment and comments. Few people fully understand the principles of Reflexology and imagination is a powerful tool. The therapist should always be professional and ethical in his/her approach to work, especially in answering clients' questions with regard to areas or organs being worked on.

Should a professional Reflexologist feel that the client being treated would benefit by seeking medical advice, or that he/she should be referred to a therapist with different or more appropriate skills; then the professional Reflexologist is both morally and ethically bound to give this advice to his/her client.

# ABNORMALITIES OF THE FEET THAT AFFECT OTHER REFLEX ZONES

1.  Infected toe nails normally indicate that the Reflex Zones to the Head Area have been affected.

2.  Hammer Toes and similar deformities suggest the Head and Face Zones are or have been affected.

3.  Flat feet would indicate the Reflex Zones to the Spinal Column are affected.

4.  Congestion in the ankle and or heel area would indicate affected Reflex Zones in the Pelvis and Hip Joint.

5.  Bunions. (Hallux Vulgus) suggests congestion in the Reflex Zones of the Cervical Spine.

6.  Corns showing anywhere on the feet indicates that the Reflex Zone to that area might be affected. If the corn presents itself in the shoulder reflex point or similar area this would naturally tell us that there might well be a problem in the shoulder area.

7.  Athletes Foot. (Tinea Pedis) Observe carefully. The spread of the infection may cover more than one zone. When there is infection present or there is a change of colour or texture radiating from that area it usually indicates an underlying problem in the affected zones.
    If athletes foot is present or if there is any doubt work on the client's hands but do examine the feet first.

8.  I believe that any change in the skeletal, muscular or tissue structure of the foot will, like the athletes foot, suggest an underlying problem in the corresponding organ of the body. Therefore even if the client does not complain of problems within an area where we get visible signs of such, it is still worthwhile to concentrate on those areas even if the skin is thick. Eventually we should get results. Alternatively instead of working on areas of hard skin work on the corresponding area on the hand after you have completed the foot routine. (Never break from the foot routine to treat the hand).

# TIMING YOUR TREATMENTS

The professional therapist is not treating people only because he or she believes in what they are doing but also in order to make their living. Therefore it is of great importance to get oneself well organised at the beginning of the day.

I always make a one and a half hour appointment for a client on their first visit. This allows me to give a consultation and deal with any unexpected eventuality that might arise on the first day. It is extremely difficult to be precise in timing treatments thereafter; so for this reason it is best to allow one hour for every client. I work on the premise of ten minutes for preparation; five at the beginning and end of each treatment.

Some clients can take and indeed some need, a full treatment of forty to forty-five minutes. Yet there is the client who is so sensitive that five or ten minutes is all they can endure without a break, especially on a first or second visit.
Always allow the client a break from discomfort during a treatment. Don't just plod on regardless of reactions.
To continue to treat a sensitive crystal laden foot for a longer period of time than the person can effectively cope with will result in there being too many toxins being released into the blood stream and this can result in making the client feel ill and tired; completely defeating the object of the exercise.

# CHILDREN

When dealing with children it is wise to make sure that the parent or guardian is aware of the limitations of the treatment. Never treat children for longer than five minutes in the very young and at no time or age for longer than fifteen minutes.

Treatment on the very young is like stroking and on the older child it is necessary to use only the finger and not the thumb. The therapist must use discretion with regard to timing when dealing with all clients, however this is even more important when dealing with children.

**It is important to note that it is a legal requirement as well as an ethical obligation to seek medical assistance for any undiagnosed conditions in children. Do not attempt to treat anything that may need medical attention.**

## THE ELDERLY

It might be necessary to take a little longer with these people. They cannot move quickly and while the therapist would naturally offer help where it is needed, it is not kind or professional to rush the less able.

## THE DIABETIC CLIENT (SEE PAGE 23 - 'CAUTION').
This condition requires careful treatment.

It is important for the therapist to keep to time as most people have busy schedules.

# HOW TO DECIDE ON THE TREATMENT

All clients should benefit from a course of eight treatments usually performed on a weekly basis.

Many clients like to maintain contact with the therapist on a monthly basis after the initial course.

Many clients just require a 'one off' pick-me-up treatment.

All treatments should consist of a complete Reflexology routine. During this pressure massage, when a reaction is felt the therapist should stop and treat that specific area seven times (in other words, seven distinct pressure circles). When the routine is completed the therapist should return to all the areas that needed extra treatment and repeat on each of these areas the seven pressure circles.

When the client is very sensitive treat with three pressure circles each time and not seven.

Occasionally one will meet a client whose foot is so crystal laden or they are so sensitive that the treatment would be most beneficially performed on the basis of commencing with one or two pressure circles and then increasing gradually on each visit until seven pressure circles can be tolerated.

Many good therapists never break from this routine throughout their lives. It is a very good principle to which all student therapists should adhere.

# REACTIONS TO REFLEXOLOGY (SECTION 1)

These can be broken into two types of reaction and the client can have these reactions explained to them as part of the consultation.

1    Those reactions that happen during treatment.

2    Those that happen after your treatment.

# SOME OF THE REACTIONS THAT MIGHT HAPPEN DURING TREATMENT

A feeling of being very cold.
(care should be taken not to give any heavy pressures and the circle pressures should be reduced to two; gradually increasing the number with successive treatments)

Changes in expression.

Crying, groaning, laughing, sighing, or singing.

Gestures of pain.

Profuse sweating on the palms of the hands.

Visible contraction of the muscles.

**To calm and relax the client**
Speak in a calm voice while gently effleuraging the whole foot, the effleurage can be alternated with a solar plexus massage or just stop and hold.

The therapist should also be aware that reactions unrelated to Reflexology could well occur in the clinic; for example, a heart attack or asthmatic attack. It is for this reason I think it advisable that all practicing therapists who are not medically qualified should hold a valid Certificate in First Aid.

# REACTIONS TO REFLEXOLOGY (SECTION 2)

# REACTIONS OCCURRING BETWEEN TREATMENT SEQUENCES

These can sometimes involve temporary discomfort or pain.

Increase in urination.

Increase in bulk volume and frequency of the stool.

Increase in nasal secretions.

Increase of, or the appearance of vaginal discharge.

Toothache, usually due to tooth decay or gum infections.

Feeling very tired.

Feeling very sleepy.

Feeling wonderful.

Clients will also explain how, for example, they caught a cold last week after they had received a treatment. They will sometimes go on to express their fears of getting a cold etc., if they have more treatments. It is worthwhile taking the time to explain to the client that all illness is preceded by an incubation period which may last for days or much longer before the illness becomes apparent.

All clients who react in an unusual way or give the therapist grounds to suspect a serious illness must be referred to their own doctor. The therapist can always contact the client's doctor by letter explaining his/her fears.

( clients consent is required ). The therapist may also ask the doctor for advice as to whether treatment can be continued or if it would be wiser to terminate the treatments during medical investigation. A sample of such a letter will be found on page 55.

Doctors may react in different ways to this type of letter both favourably and unfavourably. Some have been known to ask for a fee. However I am delighted to say that the majority of doctors I hear about are only too pleased to see therapists behaving in a caring and professional manner. All letters sent to a doctor which necessitate a reply should, as a matter of common courtesy, have a stamped addressed envelope enclosed.

# PERSONAL HYGIENE

Take a daily bath or shower.

Prevent body odour by using a deodorant.

Use a mouthwash to prevent bad breath.

Clean teeth twice daily. Have regular dental checks.

Have a clean handkerchief in case of the necessity to cough or sneeze and please use it when necessary. Do not sneeze or cough over others.

Wear clean clothes and underwear daily.

Don't forget the socks, stockings or tights. They need changing at least once a day.

Keep hair clean and tidy. Make sure it does not fall onto your face when your head is bent as this can obscure the client's view; most people would prefer to see our faces when talking to us.

Keep nails short and, like the whole hand, impeccably clean.

Wash hands before and after each treatment.

Wash hands after using the toilet.

Wear a clean uniform or coat. It looks professional.

Wear clean shoes.

You must be able to take care of yourself before you attempt to take care of others.

You are offering a personal service where you are in very close proximity to others and your odour can be offensive to them. So if you smoke, drink or enjoy spicy food remember the smell can linger not just on your breath but on your clothes as well.

It is also worth bearing in mind that perfumes and aftershaves need to be used sparingly. The client might not share your love for a particular make or brand.

# HYGIENE AT WORK

Hygiene is of the utmost importance in any treatment. When dealing with feet it is worth bearing in mind that the possibility of infection and contagion is always present. Conditions such as Athletes Foot (tinea Pedis), fungal infections of the nail and verruca (a flat wart) are but a few.

1.  The therapist's hands must be washed before and after each client.

2.  A paper towel should be used to dry the feet.

3.  Rest client's feet on a paper towel during treatment.

4.  Cover knee and footrest with tissue. If tissue is not used then the covers must be changed after each client and washed before any further use.

5.  Application of all solutions to the feet should be with cotton wool or tissue. A clean cotton wool or tissue to be used for each foot.

6.  Sterilize bowl with liquid disinfectant after each use. All disposable material should be placed in a pedal bin immediately after use.

7.  Have a pair of plastic gloves nearby for emergencies.

8.  Always read consultation card just prior to client's arrival to refresh your memory and always complete details of treatment on the card immediately the client leaves or while he/she is getting ready to leave. Never put off this task until the end of the day or until you see "just one more client".

9.  At the end of the day waste should be burned if possible or placed in a plastic bag and sealed ready for refuse collection.

10. Make sure working area is clean and surroundings pleasant.

11. Do not smoke or allow client to smoke during treatment.

# THE THERAPIST AT WORK

Reflexology is an art. This art, like all other forms of art, will take time and a lot of practice to master. The student will soon realize this is not a subject that can be easily learned from a book. However, if it is not possible to receive tuition immediately, carefully follow the instructions and diagrams in this book as well as paying special attention to the suggested routine. I would, however, strongly advise all students thinking of working in the profession of Reflexology to take a qualifying course before working as a public practitioner.

Reflexology is not a cure for all ills, although this ancient therapy will help most people.

Before the treatment prepare a consultation card. (An example of such a card is given on page 50).

Check there are no contra-indications (reason why treatment cannot or should not be performed). There is a comprehensive list of precautions and contra-indications (pages 21 and 23).

Explain Reflexology to the client. Keep it brief. Some people are very interested and will want to know more. In this case then, of course, do explain but do not fall into the trap of trying to explain all you know about the therapy at that moment. There is plenty of time during the treatment to chat.

When working it is necessary to use both hands; one to hold the foot or hand steady, the other to do the work.

Once again I have broken with tradition here and have not found it necessary to follow the theory or practice laid down by some, that it is obligatory to treat the left foot with the left hand and the right foot with the right hand. As a teacher I soon realized that not all my pupils were as dexterous as myself; so over the years I myself practised using my hands in all combinations imaginable and found the success of my treatments to be the same as when I performed the treatment using the corresponding hand. I now believe and teach that if the therapist finds working with one hand more comfortable than working with the other then he/she should work in this manner. Most Reflexology is performed using the basic thumb and finger technique. Work over the reflex area using the first joint of the thumb or finger not the whole digit. Many people believe that to use the inside or medial aspect of the digit is preferable to using the ball or tip.

The movement used in Reflexology is like bowing the first joint of the thumb or index finger up and down while making a slow movement over the reflex area. This movement has been likened to the movement of a caterpillar.

# POSITION FOR WORKING

The comfort of both therapist and client is of equal importance for the completion of an enjoyable treatment. When the professional therapist works he or she uses the standard couch or therapy chair, but if the treatment is being given in the home then an armchair can be used for the client but the lower legs and feet should be raised and supported. I have found that the padded adjustable garden chair (lounger) is the nearest to the ideal therapy chair.

In cold weather use a blanket to keep the client warm during treatment.

The therapist should sit at a comfortable distance from the client's feet which should not necessitate the arms to be fully outstretched.

The treatment commences with a relaxing foot massage. It is during this massage that the therapist gets his/her first impression of the feet, noting temperature, colour, bone structure and condition of the skin.

It is important not to lay the client flat. When working in the clinic situation use the couch/ chair backrest for support. In the home or hospital situation place one or two cushions/pillows under the head. Both methods will enable the client to see the therapist at work. This offers a measure of security and helps in building a relationship of trust. This position also gives the therapist the opportunity to observe the client's facial expressions and reactions, whether they be those of pain or relaxation, and therefore the treatment can be altered accordingly.

# SOME JOINT LOOSENING EXERCISES TO PRACTISE BEFORE YOU START WORK

1   Stand with outstretched arms in front. Open and close hands ten times (10).

2   Stand still holding arms outstretched as in the previous movement. Bend hand up and down from wrist ten times slowly, ten times fast.

3   Extend the arms to the side. Rotate wrist rapidly in a clockwise direction ten times. Repeat the movement in an anti-clockwise direction ten times.

4   Remain standing. Extend arms out to the side and push backwards twice. Bring arms to the front. Stretch out and push forward twice. Repeat complete movement ten times.

5   Stretch arms out in front, fingers pointing straight ahead, little finger side of hand towards floor, thumb toward ceiling. Hold fingers slightly apart. Now move hand from wrist up and down slowly at first gradually getting faster.

6   Stretch arms out in front. Close hand into fist, thumb on outside. Now throw your hands open. Repeat ten times.

7   Sit down and relax for a few minutes then bring your hands across in front of you. Close fingers into palm but leave thumb free. Try to make your thumbs bow to each other by bending the first joint (joint nearest nail). Repeat ten times.

8   Remain seated and this time try the movement by using your index finger (finger next to thumb) and remember to repeat ten times.

The next exercise to try is the Reflexology movement. Get a volunteer to let you practise on the feet. If there is not one around you can try this on your own hand.

1    Find the waist line area. Slide the thumb slowly across this line; lift and return to starting point.

2    This time move across in a slide-stop, slide-stop movement and then lift and return to start point.

3    Slide and stop as before only this time press ball and tip of thumb into foot (or hand). This will raise the first joint, (be careful not to dig your thumb nail into the flesh). Hold this position for a second, relax thumb and slide a fraction. Repeat movement. Continue this slide, press, raise until you reach the other side, then start all over again. Work thumb away from you if possible.

4    When you feel fairly confident with this movement using your thumb change to the index finger and repeat all of the movement in exactly the same way. Once again try to work moving index finger away from you all the time.

When you have mastered the art of bending the joint in the practise sessions across the foot, you can practise up and down the foot from heel to toe. Your aim is eventually to be able to walk across or up and down with little or no discomfort to you. Do not overdo this joint bending, as you might well have to pay the price the next day with aches and pains.

One other movement to practise is the webbing pinch. This is basically pinching between the toes. Place the index finger on top of the foot on the webbing and the thumb underneath the toes on the webbing. Grip the webbing between the fingers. A word of warning, this can be a very painful area so be very gentle.

The preceding movements are the main movements of Reflexology , however there are two further movements used by some therapists.

1.    The Rotation. In this movement the thumb is placed on a painful area and the foot or hand is rotated.

2.    The Hooking technique. The thumb is pressed very deeply into the flesh on the reflex point then used like a hook kept in place and the flesh pulled to one side. It is mainly used on the heel area due to the thickness of the flesh.

# IS IT NECESSARY TO GIVE A BOWL OF WATER? IS IT NECESSARY TO USE OILS AND CREAMS?

Reflexology is a treatment always performed on clean feet. Offensive odour may cause embarrassment to both therapist and client alike. The client will not relax and enjoy a treatment if they feel that you, the therapist, are being subject to unpleasant smells or excessively sweaty feet.

It is a good idea to offer a bowl of water to those clients who have not had a chance to take a shower or bath for some time. A building worker, for example, who has been in his shoes and socks all day is likely to sweat more than the average housewife. The water used should not contain chemical additives or perfume. A few drops of blended Aromatherapy Oil (e.g. Lavender or Lemon) or some Salt or Cider Vinegar is acceptable just to refresh. The water must not be hot as this will heat the feet artificially and as a result circulation will be increased. Further Reflexology may over stimulate and result in the treatment being less effective than it might otherwise be.

For those clients who do not need a bowl of water the feet can be refreshed by wiping with a pad soaked in a refreshing solution i.e. Tonic, Witch Hazel or Surgical Spirit.

It is important to give a Reflexology Treatment on dry feet or hands. This gives the opportunity to feel and work deeply without the hands sliding over the flesh. It is for this reason I always dry the feet thoroughly after the cleaning or refreshing process. Some therapists like to use an Aromatherapy Oil or Cream, especially on dry or problem feet. I can see no reason why this oil or cream cannot be applied at the end of the Reflexology part of the treatment and the final massage performed with it.

NOTE. Aromatherapy oil should always be blended by a qualified Aromatherapist before being used by a Reflexologist.

The therapist is in a position to advise the client of the benefits of bathing the feet daily and of the necessity to change socks or tights at least once a day in order to keep feet fresh and healthy. Exercise tact and thoughtfulness when giving such advice.

In the case of excessively sweaty feet the client should be advised to soak their feet as often as possible in a bowl of warm water to which has been added some lemon juice or vinegar. Better still would be to use a few drops of blended Aromatherapy Essential Oil in the bath or foot bowl. These oils should be purchased from a professional Aromatherapist.

# THE FIRST PAIR OF FEET

# I HAVE NO ONE TO TEACH ME REFLEXOLOGY

The first pair of feet are always the most frightening to begin work on. So the first thing to do is to learn client preparation, contra indications, precautions, hand exercise, the three transverse lines on the diagram, notes on hygiene and the foot massage.

Practise the foot massage movements on your own hand. This way at least you can learn the Step by Step routine which can remove some of the anguish when you come to a practical situation.

Find a friend or member of the family who would enjoy having a relaxing foot massage and would be patient while you practise you hand holds for giving the reflexology treatment.

The first few practise sessions could be very simple and easy. There is no need at this stage to know which organ of the body is represented where on the foot; just follow these simple instructions and diagrams. When you have mastered this routine then it is time to progress to the full Reflexology routine.

Prepare the client with feet raised. Make yourself comfortable and begin.

When you have completed the massage hold the foot steady with one hand and work up and down all the toes underneath and on the sides.

Next step is to use one hand to bend the toes back very gently and with the free hand (thumb) work from below the pad on the sole of the foot (diaphragm line -see diagram B -page 11) to the base of the toes. Cover the whole area, working upwards, returning to the diaphragm line each time. If you find it difficult to work up then work backwards and forwards across the area.

Move to the narrow part of the foot or waist line (see diagram B -page 11). Work up from the waist line to the diaphragm line in exactly the same manner as for the previous area. When you are satisfied that you have covered that area move down to the next line, the pelvic floor line, and repeat your movement from this line up to the waist line or across from Z 1 to Z 5.

Move down to tip of heel and work over the hard heel pad up to the pelvic floor line or across from Z 1 to Z 5. This movement can be alternated working from Z 5 to Z 1.

Lift the heel slightly and return it to rest in the palm of one of your hands. With the other hand stroke up the back and sides of the leg from heel to knee for as high as you can reach.

Next movement is to support the heel as before and with the thumb of the other hand work down the edge or side of the foot from the big toe to the heel, returning to start point and repeating the process (following the curve of the bone).

Change hands. This time work in the same manner but work from the edge of the foot on the little toe side to heel, returning to start point and repeating the process (follow the curve of the bone).

Work on toes on the top of the foot from nail to base; then work from base of toes towards the heel and the leg, work around the ankle area.

When working on the top and sides of the foot either work up and down or across the area whichever is more comfortable. The important thing is to have a method and a routine to follow.

# CONSULTATION CARD

| | |
|---|---|
| Name | Dr's Name |
| Address | Address |
| Tel No. | Tel No. |
| D.O.B | |
| Occupation | Your Height |
| Reason for Visit | Your Weight |
| Referred By | |

## MEDICAL HISTORY

Medication to include Birth Control Pill or Hormone Replacement Therapy

Illnesses : Chicken Pox   Glandular Fever   Shingles   Mumps   Measles
Polio   Rubella   Scarlet Fever.

Operations

Accidents, injuries or falls with approximate dates
Back Problems

General State of Health
Do you or any member of your family suffer with any problems related to the following?
Diabetes,  Epilespsy,  Blood Pressure (H/L), Thrombosis, Heart,  Chest,
Migraine,  Kidneys,  Bladder,  Digestion, Varicose Veins,  Allergies,
Hepatitis. Hay fever,  Asthma
Skin Problems.

Are you Pregnant?

Do you have regular Periods?

Date of last Period?

Do you suffer with Premenstrual Tension?
Last visit to Doctor. Reason?

Have you been to hospital for X-Ray or tests during the last three years?
Date                                    Therapist

50

DO YOU ?

Smoke _____ How many daily _____
Drink alcohol _____ Daily _____ Weekly _____ Infrequently _____
Drink          Tea _____ Coffee _____ How many daily _____
Drink          Water_____ How many glasses daily _____
Drink          Other liquids _____ How many glasses daily _____
Have a balanced diet _____ Eat regular meals _____
Eat before going to bed _____ Eat between meals _____
Take exercise _____ Daily ____ Weekly _____ Infrequently ____ Never _____
Work hours          Regular_____ Flexi_____ Shift _____ Unspecified ____
Take care of children _____ How many _____ Ages _____
Take care of the Elderly _____ Sick_____ Handicapped _____
Sleep          Well_____ Poorly_____ Restlessly _____
Do you suffer from DEPRESSION/TENSION/ANXIETY/STRESS_____
How does the above condition affect you _____
_____
_____
Is your outlook optimistic _____ pessimistic_____
Do you have any physical handicap _____
Do you wear glasses/contact lenses or hearing aid _____
POSTURE          Straight_____ Rounded shoulders _____
PERSONALITY          Confident _____ Nervous_____ Mixture _____

|  | RIGHT FOOT | LEFT FOOT |
|---|---|---|
| Colour |  |  |
| Texture |  |  |
| Muscle Tone |  |  |
| Flat Foot |  |  |
| High Arch |  |  |
| Skin Condition |  |  |
| Hard Skin Build up. |  |  |
| Area |  |  |
| Zone |  |  |
| Skeletal Deformities |  |  |

# THE REASON FOR THE CONSULTATION CARD

Through question and answer the therapist is able to ascertain if the client is suffering with any contagious of infectious conditions or indeed if there are any contra indications. A carefully recorded consultation card will help to build a picture of the client's general state of health.

# THE TREATMENT CARD

This card gives the therapist the opportunity to record accurately, allowing him/her to build a quick reference system as well as a complete picture of the client's progress.

All therapists should keep accurate records of treatments.

## A SAMPLE
## TREATMENT CARD

| DATE | R.F. | L.F. | REACTIONS | TIME | SIG |
|---|---|---|---|---|---|
| 16/5/91 | Sinuses C | Sinuses S | Very sensitive to touch. Pulled both feet away | 10am | |

C = CRYSTAL     S= SENSITIVITY     SIG= SIGNATURE
OF THERAPIST

The reverse of treatment card can be used to build a case history of the client.

# CASE HISTORY

# RENÉE TANNER
# REFLEXOLOGIST
# M.I.F.R.

Doctor S. Jones

11 Some Street
Croydon                        1st June 1987

Dear Doctor Jones,
re: Mrs Mary Jane White, 00 Central Road, Croydon.

Your patient, my client, Mrs. M.J. White, has come to me for a Reflexology
Treatment massage.

In view of the fact that she has had a recent operation and you are familiar
with her condition, I would be grateful for your permission to carry out this
treatment.
Would you please sign the endorsement at the foot of this letter and with any
comments return it to me.

For your convenience I have enclosed a stamped addressed envelope for your
reply.

Yours faithfully,


Renée Tanner

78 Walkers Road, Croydon CR0 1OO     Tel:
...........................................................................................................................
I Dr Jones.................................................................give my permission for
Mrs Mary J White to receive a Reflexology Massage.

Signed.................................................................

Dated.................................................................
Return to: Renée Tanner, 78 Walkers Road, Croydon CR0 1OO

55

# A SUGGESTED METHOD FOR REFLEXOLOGY TREATMENT

1   Prepare Client Record Card and confirm as far as possible that there are no Contra Indications

2   Make Client Comfortable

3   Cleanse and Dry both Feet

4   Give a relaxing Foot Massage to both feet. - Starting on right foot.

5   Perform Reflexology Treatment starting on right foot

6   Give a Foot Massage to both feet. - Starting on right foot.

7   Wash your Hands

8   Make a Further Appointment if deemed to be necessary

9   Complete Treatment Card

# TREATMENT TYPES

Two types of treatment are referred to in Reflexology

    1. SYMPTOMATIC TREATMENT
    2. CASUAL TREATMENT.

Symptomatic treatment as the name suggests deals with the symptom. This is the type of treatment used in self help situations.
The way it works : - If someone has a pain in the head then the treatment is given to the reflex point of the head. Someone with stomach pains is treated only in the reflex area of the stomach.

Casual treatment is the type of treatment performed by the therapist seeking the underlying cause of the symptom. Therefore the entire foot receives a Reflexology treatment with the sensitive or crystal areas being given specific treatment.
For example the client complaining of headache might well be found to have a disorder in any of the five zones.
The client with stomach pains may be found to have reactions in the reflex areas of the stomach, intestines, lower back, solar plexus, etc...

In the main the qualified therapist will use this latter form of therapy.

# MASSAGE ROUTINE

# MASSAGE PRIOR TO AND ON COMPLETION OF A REFLEXOLOGY TREATMENT

Give client a bowl of warm water to soak feet, especially if he or she has been working all day. (This is a common courtesy to both client and therapist).

Alternatively, wipe feet with a cotton wool pad previously soaked in surgical spirit, witchazel or similar solution.

1    Place both hands on top of the foot, fingers pointing towards ankle. Slide hands down foot from toes to ankle. Gently massage around ankle in large circular movements using two middle fingers.

2    Hold foot firmly, one hand under heel and place thumb of other hand on ball of foot just below toes. Fingers of this hand should be on top of foot. Rotate foot, first in clockwise movement then in an anti-clockwise movement. (Slow movement).

# EFFLEURAGE (DIAGRAM REF. NO.1)

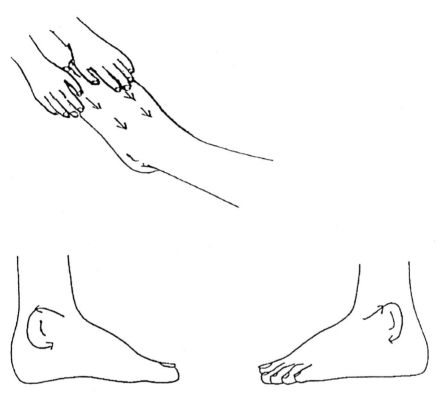

# ROTATE (DIAGRAM REF. NO.2)

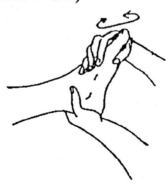

**3**    Put one hand on either side of foot, fingers pointing upwards not touching foot. Place heel of hands at either side of sole. Push inner aspect of foot (big toe side) away from you with one hand while gently pulling outer aspect towards you with other hand. A push/pull movement.

**4**    Place fingers on top of foot, thumbs underneath. Have balls of thumb flat against sole, fingers flat on top (one hand will be lower down the foot than the other). Work thumbs in a zig-zag movement from base of toes to base of heel and back (quick movement).

## PUSH PULL (DIAGRAM REF. NO. 3)

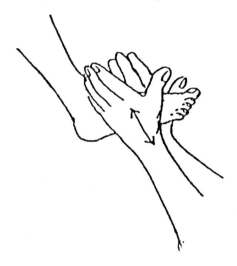

## ZIG ZAG (DIAGRAM REF. NO.4)

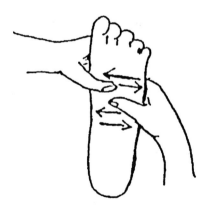

5     Hold foot on either side, heel of hand (wrist side) towards toes, fingers towards ankle.  Work fingers all around ankle area.

6     Hold foot with one hand. With heel of other hand give a deep firm stroke down inner aspect (big toe side) from toe to heel.

# ANKLE MASSAGE (DIAGRAM REF. NO. 5)

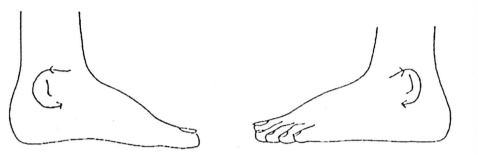

# HEEL OF HAND DOWN INSIDE FOOT (DIAGRAM REF. NO. 6)

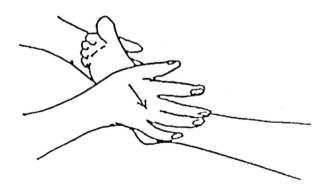

7    Put one hand on either side of foot, fingers pointing upwards not touching foot. Place heel of hands at either side of sole. Push inner aspect of foot (big toe side) away from you with one hand while gently pulling outer aspect towards you with other hand. Push pull movement ( as in movement number 3. )

8    Hold foot firmly, one hand under heel and place other hand with thumb on ball of foot just below toes. Fingers of this hand should be on top of foot. Rotate foot, firstly in a clockwise movement then in an anti-clockwise movement. (Slow movement).

## PUSH PULL (DIAGRAM REF. NO. 7)

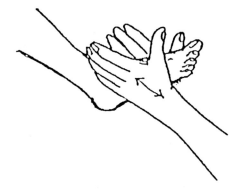

## ROTATE (DIAGRAM REF. NO. 8)

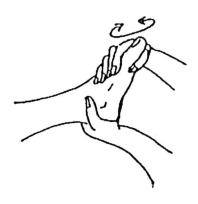

**9**     Place hands in position as for movement number 4.  Slide down sole to heel.  Firmly grip foot and pull upwards from heel towards toes.  (All pulling pressure is on sole not top of foot, as this would hurt).  Spread toes gently. Slide fingers from toe to toe allowing toes to fall back into place themselves.

**10**     Hold toes with one hand and bend them away from you (just a little); place the thumb of the free hand in position just below (on big toe side) and using the thumb work with caterpillar like movements across the foot towards the little toe side.

Change hands and repeat movement in the opposite direction.

## PULL UP HEEL TO TOE, SPREAD TOES
## (DIAGRAM REF. NO. 9)

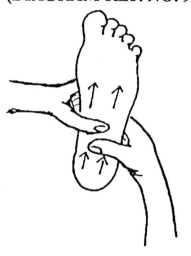 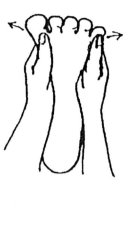

## DIAPHRAGM LINE
## (DIAGRAM REF. NO. 10)

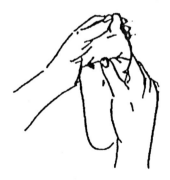

# REFLEXOLOGY ROUTINE

# RIGHT FOOT

# TREATMENT ON RIGHT FOOT

## 1. DIAPHRAGM / SOLAR PLEXUS
### Z 1 TO Z 5 AND Z 2/3

Gently push all the toes backwards with one hand. This will make the diaphragm line more visible. While holding this position use thumb of free hand to work along the diaphragm line from Z 1 to between Z 2 and 3. Stop at this point and press three times (solar plexus). Then continue to work across the foot on diaphragm line to Z 5. Then repeat the process.

## 2. HEAD AND BRAIN
### Z 1 TOE ONE

Work with the thumb from the base of the big toe (outside edge) up the outside, over the top and down the inner side (in a horseshoe shape). Return to the start point and repeat the movement. Return to the start point again, only this time work from the base of the big toe underneath to the top. Continue this movement until the base area of the big toe is treated (X 2). Now work on the top of the toe in a similar way; only this time work from the bottom of the nail to the bottom of the toe. Make sure to treat the whole area of the top of the toe X 2.

# DIAPHRAGM / SOLAR PLEXUS

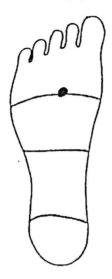

# HEAD AND BRAIN

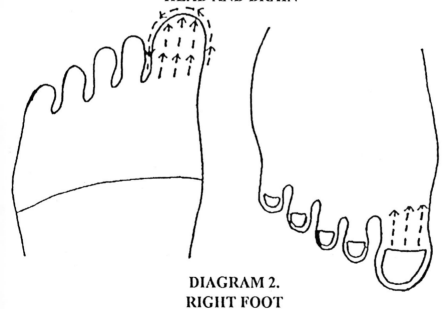

## DIAGRAM 2.
## RIGHT FOOT

## 3.   FRONT OF NECK

Put index finger at the base of the big toe; on top of the foot. Work across this base line from the outside of the toe to the inside. Stop between toe 1 and toe 2. Then return to start point and repeat the movement X 2. Making a total of three movements.

## 4.   BACK OF NECK

Work in a straight line across the base crease of the big toe (underneath). Start from outside edge. Work to inside (between toe 1 and toe 2). Return to start point and repeat X 2.

**FRONT OF NECK**

**DIAGRAM 3
RIGHT FOOT**
(Top)

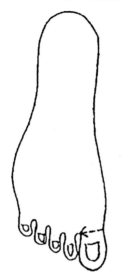

**BACK OF NECK**

**DIAGRAM 4
RIGHT FOOT**
(Sole)

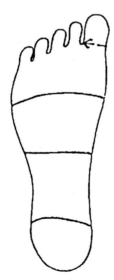

## 5.   OCCIPITAL

### Z 1 TOE ONE

Use index finger or thumb to work up inside edge of big toe (underneath ).
Start from crease line at base and make 3 very small caterpillar like
movements upwards towards top of toe.  Then stop.  Press X 3.

## 6.   EAR POINT / MASTOID PROCESS

### Z 1 TOE ONE

Work up toe for a further 3 movements then stop and press X 3.

# OCCIPITAL

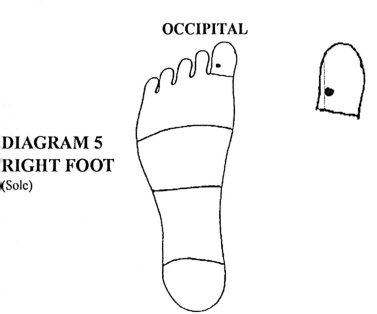

## DIAGRAM 5
## RIGHT FOOT
(Sole)

# EAR POINT - MASTOID PROCESS

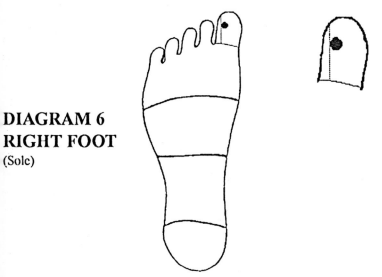

## DIAGRAM 6
## RIGHT FOOT
(Sole)

# 7.   PITUITARY

## Z 1 TOE ONE

Place thumb in centre of pad on the big toe.  Press X 3.
N.B.  When treating the male client who suffers from Acne type skin
conditions press and release X 3 again.

# 8.   SINUSES

## Z 2 TO Z 5. FOUR TOES

Work with  thumb or index finger from the base of the toe up and over the top
in a horseshoe shape (as on big toe ).  Then work with thumb from base of toe
to the top of the toe X 1.  Work once more from base of toe to the bulb, lift the
bulb and roll it back gently.  Repeat on all four toes. ( 2 to 5 )
N.B.  The area of the cranial nerves will also be found on the side of the toes

**PITUITARY**

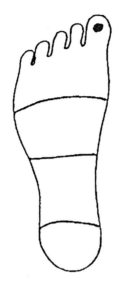

**DIAGRAM 7
RIGHT FOOT**
(Sole)

**SINUSES**

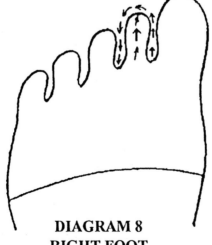

**DIAGRAM 8
RIGHT FOOT**
(Sole)

## 9.  TEETH

### Z 1 TO Z 5. FIVE TOES

This time work on top of the toes.  Start at the base of the nail and work down to the bottom of each individual toe X 2.  Do as many movements as are necessary to cover the whole area from nail to base of toe.

## 10.  LYMPHATICS OF HEAD / NECK

### Z 1 TO Z 5 BETWEEN TOES

Very gently pinch webbing between toes.

**TEETH**

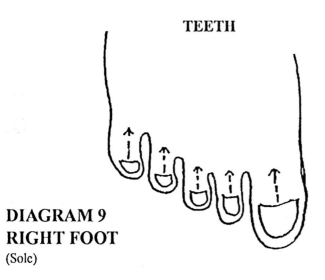

**DIAGRAM 9
RIGHT FOOT**
(Sole)

**LYMPHATICS OF HEAD / NECK**

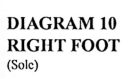

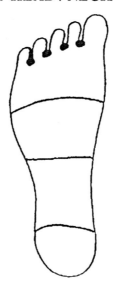

**DIAGRAM 10
RIGHT FOOT**
(Sole)

## 11.  EYES / EARS

### Z 2 TO Z 5 UNDER TOES

Bend toes back gently with thumb of free hand.  Work on top part of exposed pad along the top of the ridge at the base of the toes.  Work from Z 2 to Z 5 X 2.

 Note, eyes under Z 2/3 and ears under Z 4/5.

## 12.  EYE POINT

### Z 2/3 UNDER TOES

Use thumb or index finger to press down firmly on the pad at the base of the toes (sole) between Z 2 and Z 3.  ( Do not press into toes )

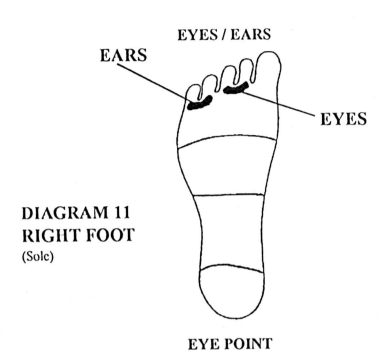

EYES / EARS

EARS

EYES

**DIAGRAM 11
RIGHT FOOT**
(Sole)

EYE POINT

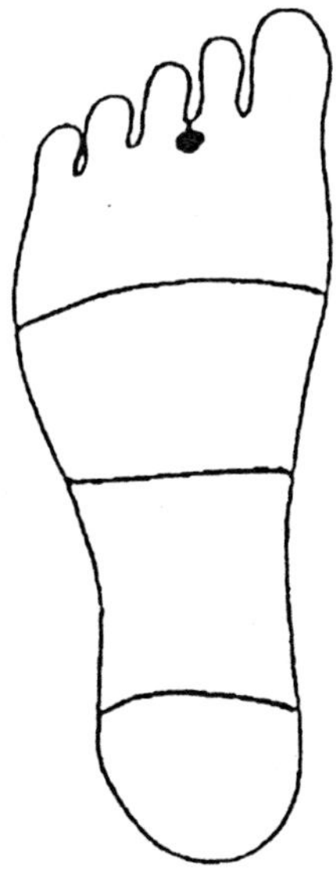

**DIAGRAM 12
RIGHT FOOT**
(Sole)

## 13.  EAR POINT

### Z 4/5 UNDER TOES

Use thumb or index finger to press down firmly on the pad at the base of toes (sole) between Z 4 and Z 5.  ( Do not press into toes )

## 14.  EUSTACHIAN TUBE

### Z 3/4/ UNDER TOES

Put the index finger of one hand at the base of the toes between Z 3 and Z 4 on the top of the foot.  Put the thumb of the same hand on the sole at the base of the toes (on the pad) between Z 3 and Z 4.  Press down firmly while pinching together gently.  This hold is on the fleshy area not on or between the toes.

**EAR POINT**

**DIAGHRAM 13**
**RIGHT FOOT**
(Solc)

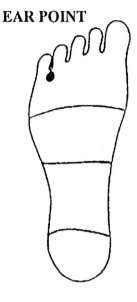

**EUSTACHIAN TUBE**

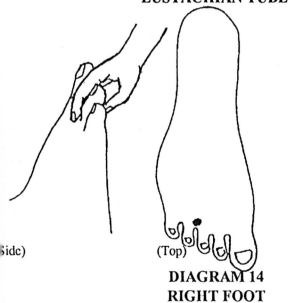

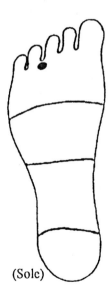

(Sidc)

(Top)

(Solc)

**DIAGRAM 14**
**RIGHT FOOT**

## 15.  BALANCE

### Z 4 TOE FOUR

Slide index finger down toe 4 on top from nail to base; then press into base X 2.

## 16.  SHOULDER POINT / LYMPHATICS
### Z 4/5 TOP OF FOOT AND SOLE

Use index finger to slide down from base of the toe on top of foot for about half an inch, or until small hollow is felt. Put thumb of same hand on corresponding point on the sole of the foot. Now press firmly and release X 2. Hold thumb and index finger in grip position. Now work with a circular movement in the area of the shoulder whilst maintaining grip. **To do this movement the working hand can take its position either from the side of the foot or over the top as in diagram opposite.**

**BALANCE**

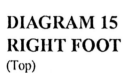

**DIAGRAM 15
RIGHT FOOT**
(Top)

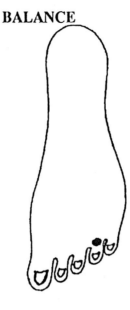

**SHOULDER POINT**

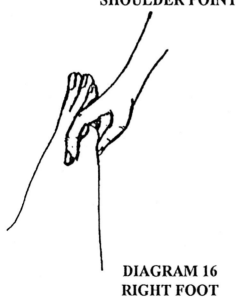

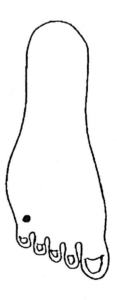

**DIAGRAM 16
RIGHT FOOT**

## 17.   THYROID / PARATHYROID / THYMUS
(general area treatment)

### Z 1 SOLE

Place the thumb on the diaphragm line at the outer edge of Z 1 toe 1.  Begin caterpillar like walk towards Z 2 but stop between Z 1 and Z 2.  Turn the thumb to point towards the toes and work up crease line to between big toe and toe 2.  Return to start point and repeat entire movement.

## 17A.THYROID

### Z 1 SOLE

Lift the thumb and place it in the centre of the pad of the ball of the foot under the big toe, move one point up towards the base of the big toe and give three pressure circles.

# THYROID / PARATHYROID / THYMUS
## (GENERAL AREA TREATMENT)

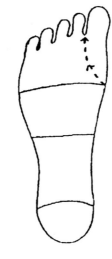

**DIAGRAM 17
RIGHT FOOT**
(Sole)

**THYROID**

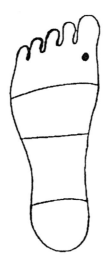

**DIAGRAM 17A
RIGHT FOOT**
(Sole)

## 17B.    PARATHYROID

Z 1 SOLE

Lift the thumb and place it in line with the thyroid on the edge of zone one (next to Z 2); move thumb one point up towards the base of the big toe and give three pressure circles.

## 17C.    THYMUS

Z 1 SOLE

Lift the thumb and place it in line with the thyroid on the ball of the foot on the sole (as close to the edge of the foot as possible while still working on the sole) and give three pressure circles.

## 18.  OESOPHAGUS / TRACHEA

Z 1 SOLE

Place the thumb on the diaphragm line at the edge of Z 1. Work from this point up to the base of the big toe. Return to diaphragm line and continue to work to base of toe until the entire pad has been treated in this way.

## PARATHYROID

**DIAGRAM 17B
RIGHT FOOT**
(Sole)

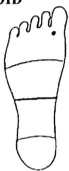

## THYMUS

**DIAGRAM 17C
RIGHT FOOT**
(Sole)

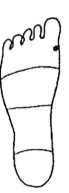

## OESOPHAGUS / TRACHEA

**DIAGRAM 18
RIGHT FOOT**
(Sole)

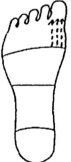

# 19. CHEST / LUNGS

## Z 2 TO Z 5 SOLE

Put thumb on diaphragm line directly under Z 2. Work from diaphragm line to base of toes. Continue to work in this manner until the entire area from Z 2 to Z 5 has been treated. Repeat movement.

N.B. This movement can be performed across all four zones but it is more usual for the professional therapist to work from the diaphragm towards the toes.

A note of interest !

When working from diaphragm line Z 5 to base of toe 5 reactions will give indications of shoulder problems. Treat with pressure circles if necessary.

# 20. CHEST / LUNGS CONTINUED

## Z 1 TO Z 5 TOP OF FOOT

This time work on top of the foot and use the index finger and not the thumb. Start at the base of Z 1, big toe, and work down towards leg to area corresponding to diaphragm line on the sole. Treat area from Z 1 to Z 5. When area has been treated return to start point and repeat movement.

# CHEST / LUNGS

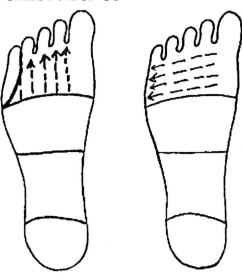

**DIAGRAM 19
RIGHT FOOT**
(Sole)

# CHEST / LUNGS - CONTINUED

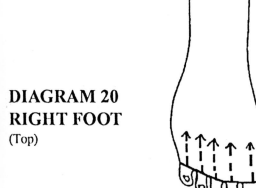

**DIAGRAM 20
RIGHT FOOT**
(Top)

## 21. UPPER ABDOMEN

### Z 1 TO Z 5 SOLE

Put thumb on waist line directly under Z 1 on the sole close to the edge of the foot. Work from waist line to diaphragm line. Continue to work in this manner until the entire area between Z 1 and Z 5 has been treated. Return to start point and repeat movement.

N.B. This movement can be performed across all five zones.

**It is more usual for the professional therapist to work across all five zones.**

## 22. GALL BLADDER (RIGHT FOOT ONLY)

### BETWEEN Z 3/4 SOLE

Put thumb on diaphragm line between Z 3 and 4. Press in and release X 2. This movement is as if the thumb is pressing up and in, under the diaphragm line. All pressure below the diaphragm line. **If you find this movement difficult try placing the tip of the thumb touching the diaphragm line and just press in.**

N.B. Massage very gently over area if gall stones are present. No pressure, as this might move the gall stones (consult Doctor).

**UPPER ABDOMEN**

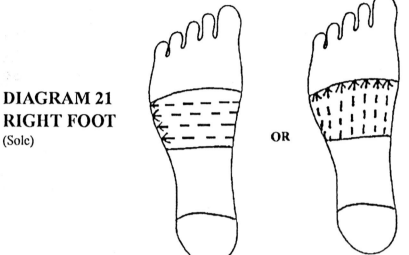

**DIAGRAM 21
RIGHT FOOT**
(Sole)

OR

**GALL BLADDER**

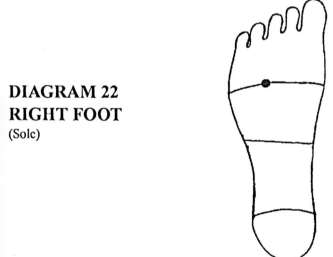

**DIAGRAM 22
RIGHT FOOT**
(Sole)

95

## 23. LIVER (RIGHT FOOT ONLY)

### Z 3 TO Z 5 SOLE

Place thumb on Z 3 just under diaphragm line. Work with thumb pointing towards Z 5 for three overlapping rows across foot from Z 3 to Z 5. Change hands. This time work from Z 5 to Z 3 in three overlapping rows.

## 24. STOMACH / PANCREAS / DUODENUM

### Z 1 TO Z 3 SOLE

Place thumb one point below diaphragm line on sole (close to edge of foot). Work from Z 1 to Z 3 across foot in three straight but overlapping rows. On completion repeat this movement working this time from Z 3 to Z 1 (change hands if necessary). While most of this area is taken up with the stomach we are also treating the duodenum/pancreas. The student of anatomy and physiology will know the area of these structures in the body. **It is necessary to exercise extreme care when dealing with a diabetic, only a gentle massage should be given by all but the very well qualified specialist/ therapist.**

**N.B. Stomach ulcers - treat with care. Very light massage over area. No pressure, as this might cause the ulcer to rupture (consult Doctor)**

# LIVER

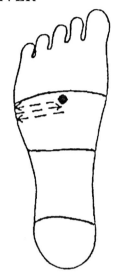

**DIAGRAM 23
RIGHT FOOT**
(Sole)

# STOMACH / PANCREAS / DUODENUM

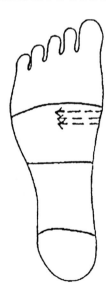

**DIAGRAM 24
RIGHT FOOT**
(Sole)

# 25. LOWER ABDOMEN / PELVIS / SMALL INTESTINE

## Z 1 TO Z 5 SOLE

Put thumb on heel pad, just below soft flesh. Work with caterpillar like movements from Z 1 to Z 5 - cover area between heel pad and waist line. When area has been treated return to start point and repeat movement.
This movement can be performed across all five zones. First working in one direction then the other. **Most professionals favour cross working for this area.**

# 26. SCIATIC LINE

## UP BACK OF LEG

Put one hand under leg, palm uppermost (against leg). Then with a slow, sliding, push movement, work from ankle up to behind the knee; return to the start point and repeat X 2. Return to start point again, this time close heel of hand onto leg in a squeezing movement, work up leg to behind knee. Return to start point and repeat X 2.

# LOWER ABDOMEN / PELVIS / SMALL INTESTINE

**DIAGRAM 25
RIGHT FOOT**
(Sole)

OR

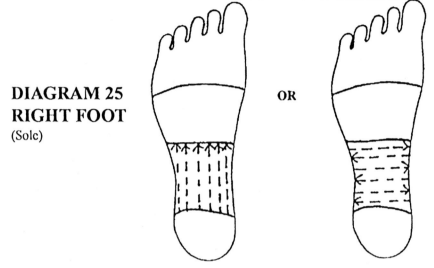

## SCIATIC LINE

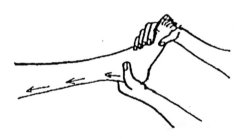

**DIAGRAM 26
RIGHT FOOT**

## 27. SCIATIC LINE - CONTINUED
## BEHIND ANKLE - ACROSS SOLE

Put thumb of one hand (pointing down towards the sole) on the soft flesh area behind the ankle bone at its highest point. Work with caterpillar like movements down behind ankle bone then across the hard heel pad on the sole of the foot (change hands if necessary) and continue to work with this movement up behind the other ankle bone to its highest point. Return to start point and repeat movement X 2. ( Total of three ).

## 28. SPINE
## INNER EDGE OF FOOT

Use the thumb to work with caterpillar like movements down inner edge of foot from just below nail area on big toe to the heel. Follow the curve of the foot (feeling for the bone). Repeat movement in opposite direction from heel to toe, then repeat entire movement.

**N.B. Due to the huge supply of nerves directly from the spinal cord to the organs of the body, treating the spine works not only on the skeletal and muscular structure of the area but gives a general treatment to the other organs of the body.**

# SCIATIC LINE - CONTINUED

(Sole)

## DIAGRAM 27
## RIGHT FOOT

(Outer side)

(Inner side)

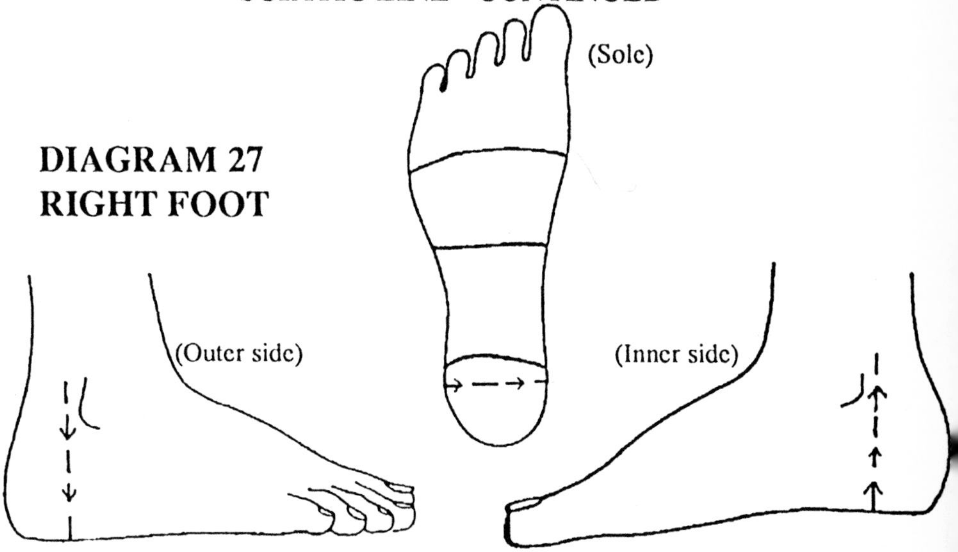

**SPINE**

## DIAGRAM 28
## RIGHT FOOT
(Sole & Medial View)

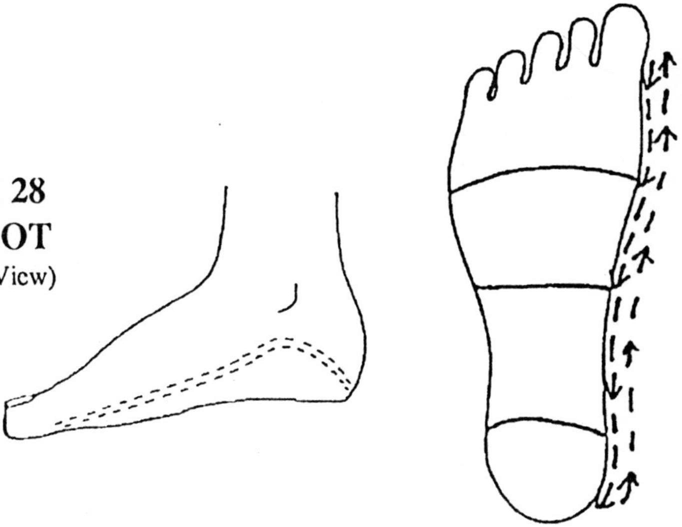

# 29.   SHOULDER / ELBOW / HIP/ KNEE / LOWER BACK

## OUTER EDGE OF FOOT

Use the thumb to work with caterpillar like movement down outer edge of the foot from below nail area on little toe to the heel.  Repeat movement in opposite direction then repeat the entire movement.

# 30.   RECTUM / ANUS / LOWER PELVIC POINT

## Z 1 TO Z 5

Put thumb on outer edge of heel in line with ankle, work with caterpillar movement around behind heel to inside corresponding area; work in a horse shoe shape (change hands if necessary).  Return to start point and repeat movement.  **This movement can be started on either the indside or the outside.**

# SHOULDER / ELBOW / HIP /KNEE / LOWER BACK

## DIAGRAM 29
## RIGHT FOOT
(Sole)

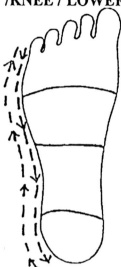

# RECTUM / ANUS LOWER PELVIC POINT

## DIAGRAM 30
## RIGHT FOOT
(Sole)

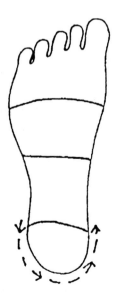

# 31.  KIDNEY / URETER TUBES

## Z 2/3

Place thumb on the waist line between Z 2 and Z 3.  Use left hand.  With tip
of thumb pointing towards toes press and release X 2.  Remove thumb, replace
thumb and press and release X 2 again.  Swivel thumb around so that tip
points towards heel, work down Z 2 to hard heel pad.  Twist hand around, still
using thumb, walk up side of foot to centre of the bladder.  Press into
centre X 2.

# 32.  BLADDER

## INNER SIDE OF FOOT

The bladder is usually visible as a slightly puffy area.  Place the thumb in the
centre of the bladder area then work in points radiating outwards. (Use small
caterpillar like movements).
**Do not work back up ureter tubes towards kidney as this may transfer any
infections present in the bladder to the kidney.**

Line 1          Work towards Z 2 toe 2 in three points
Line 2          Work towards Z 4 toe 4 in three points
Line 3          Work towards Z 5 toe 5 in three points
Line 4          Work just below line covered by line
                3 in same direction but closer to
                heel pad

# KIDNEY / URETER TUBES

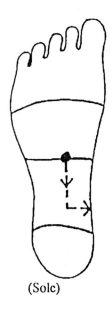

**DIAGRAM 31
RIGHT FOOT**

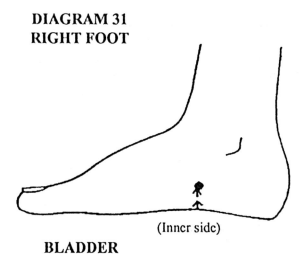

(Sole)

(Inner side)

## BLADDER

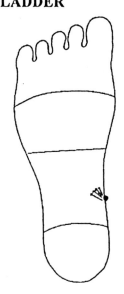

**DIAGRAM 32
RIGHT FOOT**
(Sole)

## 33. ADRENALS

Put one thumb on the kidney point pointing towards toes and bring second thumb to meet it on the big toe side. This thumb should be pointing towards the heel. Now both thumbs should be pointing in opposite directions with nails almost parallel. Remove the thumb from the kidney point. With the remaining thumb on the adrenal gland press and release gently X 3.

## 34. UTERUS / PROSTATE

### BELOW INNER ANKLE

Place index finger on inner ankle bone.
Place third finger on tip of heel.
Bend second finger slightly, it will fall in line with the other fingers. When the point of importance has been located by middle finger, remove all three fingers and place the thumb on point where the middle finger rested. Press and release X 3.
This movement can be performed with the index finger on the heel and the third finger on the ankle bone if this is found to be a more comfortable position for the therapist.
N.B. If IUD is fitted massage with great care. If any previous problems have been experienced then this area should not be treated.

**ADRENALS**

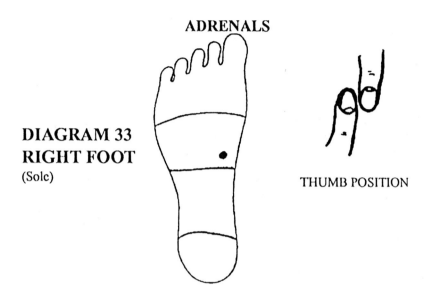

**DIAGRAM 33
RIGHT FOOT**
(Sole)

THUMB POSITION

**UTERUS / PROSTATE**

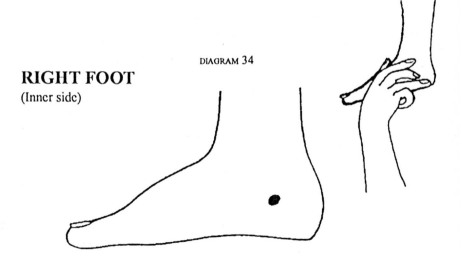

DIAGRAM 34

**RIGHT FOOT**
(Inner side)

## 35.  OVARIES / TESTES

### BELOW OUTER ANKLE

Place index finger on outer ankle bone.
Place third finger on tip of heel.
Bend second finger slightly, it will fall in line with the other fingers.  When the point of importance has been located by middle finger, remove all three fingers and place the thumb on point where the middle finger rested.  Press and release X 3.
This movement can be performed with the index finger on the heel and the third finger on the ankle bone if this is found to be a more comfortable position for the therapist.
N.B.  If the client suffers from Acne type skin conditions repeat the pressure X 3 again.


## 36.  FALLOPIAN TUBES / VAS-DEFERENCE

### TOP OF FOOT

Work with caterpillar like movement from ankle to ankle across crease line between foot and leg.  Repeat this movement in opposite direction.  Then perform the complete movement once more.

# OVARIES / TESTES

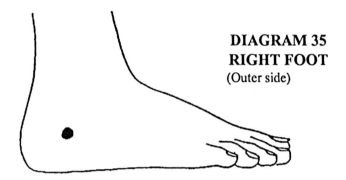

**DIAGRAM 35**
**RIGHT FOOT**
(Outer side)

# FALLOPIAN TUBES / VAS-DEFERENCE

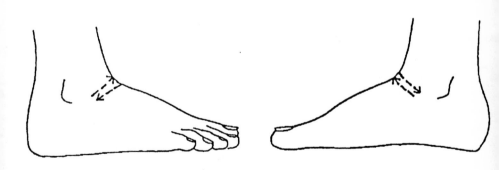

**DIAGRAM 36**
**RIGHT FOOT**

## 37. LYMPHATIC / INGUINALS / PELVIC AREA

Place the thumb on the outer edge of the heel (see diagram) pointing upwards towards the leg.
Work up behind the ankle to an area one point higher than the ankle bone, press and release X 2. Turn the thumb around so that tip is pointing towards heel, then slide the thumb back to bottom of the ankle bone. Work around the base of the bone and up in front of the ankle bone to one point higher than the bone. Press and release X 2 (horse shoe shape). Slide the thumb back to the base of the ankle bone. Next work across the leg-foot crease line to the inner ankle. **Change hands** and repeat this entire movement on the other side. Commence at the beginning again and treat the areas of both ankles including the line across the foot.

## 38. BREAST AREA
### Z 2 TO Z 5 TOP OF FOOT

Use pad of index finger to work on the top of the foot in gentle, slow, slide, press and release movement from the base of the toes to an area corresponding to the diaphragm line on the sole. Start movement at the base of toe 2, work down Z 2, work back between Z 2 and Z 3 using a gentle pull and press movement. Work each zone 2 to 5 in this manner.

# CHANGE TO LEFT FOOT

# LYMPHATICS / INGUINALS / PELVIC AREA

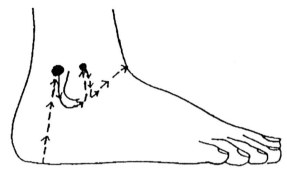

## DIAGRAM 37
## RIGHT FOOT
(Outer side)

# BREAST AREA

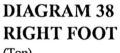

## DIAGRAM 38
## RIGHT FOOT
(Top)

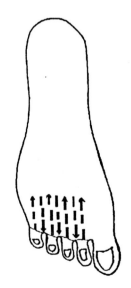

# REFLEXOLOGY ROUTINE

# LEFT FOOT

## 1.   DIAPHRAGM / SOLAR PLEXUS

### Z 1 TO Z 5 AND Z 2/3

Gently push all the toes backwards with one hand. This will make the diaphragm line more visible. While holding this position use thumb of free hand to work along the diaphragm line from Z 1 to between Z 2 and 3. Stop at this point and press three times (solar plexus). Then continue to work across the foot on diaphragm line to Z 5. Then repeat the process.

## 2.   HEAD AND BRAIN

### Z 1 TOE ONE

Work with the thumb from the base of the big toe (outside edge) up the outside, over the top and down the inner side (in a horseshoe shape). Return to the start point and repeat the movement. Return to the start point again, only this time work from the base of the big toe underneath to the top. Continue this movement until the base area of the big toe is treated (X 2). Now work on the top of the toe in a similar way; only this time work from the bottom of the nail to the bottom of the toe. Make sure to treat the whole area of the top of the toe X 2.

**DIAPHRAGM / SOLAR PLEXUS**

**DIAGRAM 1
LEFT FOOT**
(Sole)

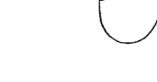

**HEAD AND BRAIN**

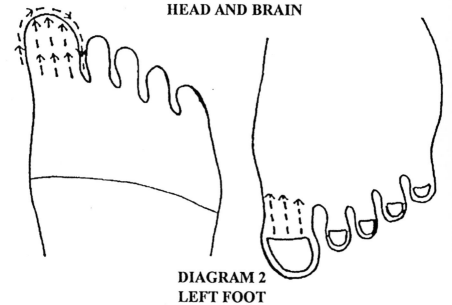

**DIAGRAM 2
LEFT FOOT**

## 3.    FRONT OF NECK

### Z 1 TOE ONE

Put index finger at the base of the big toe; on top of the foot. Work across this base line from the outside of the toe to the inside. Stop between toe 1 and toe 2. Then return to start point and repeat the movement X 2. Making a total of three movements.

## 4.    BACK OF NECK

### Z 1 TOE ONE

Work in a straight line across the base crease of the big toe (underneath). Start from outside edge. Work to inside (between toe 1 and toe 2). Return to start point and repeat X 2.

**FRONT OF NECK**

**DIAGRAM 3**
**LEFT FOOT**
(Top)

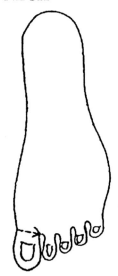

**BACK OF NECK**

**DIAGRAM 4**
**LEFT FOOT**
(Sole)

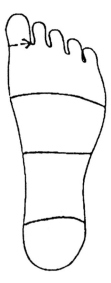

## 5.   OCCIPITAL

### Z 1 TOE ONE

Use index finger or thumb to work up inside edge of big toe (underneath ).
Start from crease line at base and make 3 very small caterpillar like
movements upwards towards top of toe.  Then stop.  Press X 3.

## 6.   EAR POINT / MASTOID PROCESS

### Z 1 TOE ONE

Work up toe for a further 3 movements then stop and press X 3.

# OCCIPITAL

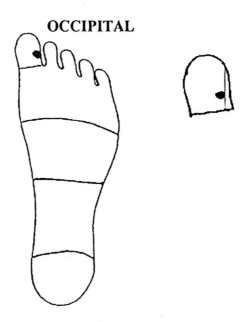

**DIAGRAM 5
LEFT FOOT**
(Sole)

# EAR POINT - MASTOID PROCESS

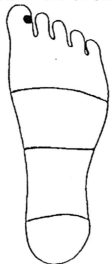

**DIAGRAM 6
LEFT FOOT**
(Sole)

## 7.　PITUITARY

### Z 1 TOE ONE

Place thumb in centre of pad on the big toe.  Press X 3.
N.B.  When treating the male client who suffers from Acne type skin
conditions press and release X 3 again.

## 8.　SINUSES

### Z 2 TO Z 5. FOUR TOES

Work with  thumb or index finger from the base of the toe up and over the top
in a horseshoe shape (as on big toe ).  Then work with thumb or index finger
from base of toes to the top of the toe X 1.  Work once more from base of toe
to the bulb, lift the bulb and roll it back gently.
N.B.  The area of the cranial nervers will also be found on the side of the toes.

**PITUITARY**

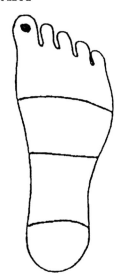

**DIAGRAM 7
LEFT FOOT**
(Sole)

**SINUSES**

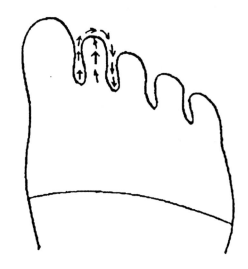

**DIAGRAM 8
LEFT FOOT**
(Sole)

## 9.   TEETH

### Z 1 TO Z 5. FIVE TOES

This time work on top of the toes.  Start at the base of the nail and work down to the bottom of each individual toe X 2.  Do as many movements as are necessary to cover the whole area from nail to base of toe.

## 10.   LYMPHATICS OF HEAD / NECK

### Z 1 TO Z 5 BETWEEN TOES

Very gently pinch webbing between toes.

# TEETH

## DIAGRAM 9
## LEFT FOOT
(Top)

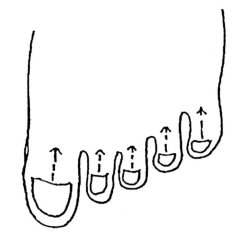

# LYMPHATICS OF HEAD / NECK

## DIAGRAM 10
## LEFT FOOT
(Sole)

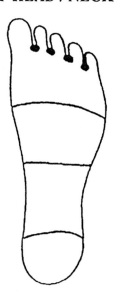

123

## 11.  EYES / EARS

Bend toes back gently with thumb of free hand.  Work on top part of exposed pad along the top of the ridge at the base of the toes.
Work from Z 2 to Z 5 X 2.  Note, eyes under Z 2/3 and ears under Z 4/5.

## 12.  EYE POINT

Use thumb or index finger to press down firmly on the pad at the base of the toes (sole) between Z 2 and Z 3.  ( Do not press into toes )

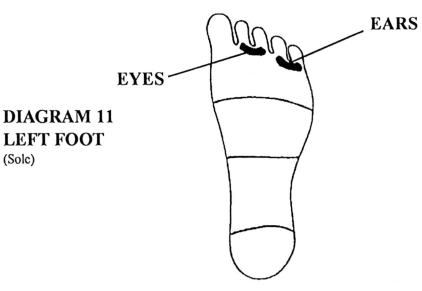

**EYES / EARS**

**EARS**

**EYES**

**DIAGRAM 11
LEFT FOOT**
(Sole)

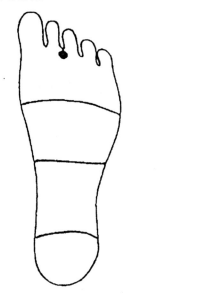

**EYE POINT**

**DIAGRAM 12
LEFT FOOT**
(Sole)

## 13.   EAR POINT

### Z 4/5 UNDER TOES

Use thumb or index finger to press down firmly on the pad at the base of toes (sole) between Z 4 and Z 5.  ( Do not press into toes )

## 14.   EUSTACHIAN TUBE

### Z 3/4 UNDER TOES

Put the index finger of one hand at the base of the toes between Z 3 and Z 4 on the top of the foot.  Put the thumb of the same hand on the sole at the base of the toes (on the pad) between Z 3 and Z 4. Press down firmly while pinching together gently.  This hold is on the fleshy area not on or between the toes.

## DIAGRAM 13
## LEFT FOOT
(Sole)

**EAR POINT**

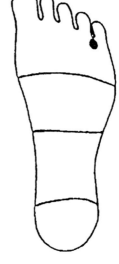

**EUSTACHIAN TUBE**

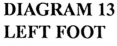

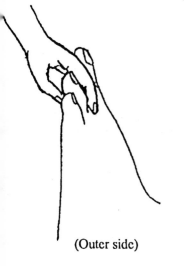

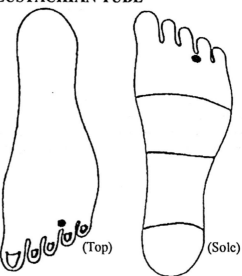

(Outer side)

(Top)

(Sole)

## DIAGRAM 14
## LEFT FOOT

127

## 15. BALANCE

### Z 4 TOE FOUR

Slide index finger down toe 4 on top from nail to base; then press into base X 2.

## 16. SHOULDER POINT / LYMPHATICS
### Z 4/5 TOP OF FOOT AND SOLE

Use index finger to slide down from base of the toe on top of foot for about half an inch, or until small hollow is felt. Put thumb of same hand on corresponding point on the sole of the foot. Now press firmly and release X 2. Hold thumb and index finger in grip position. Now work with a circular movement in the area of the shoulder whilst maintaining grip. **To do this movement the working hand can take its position either from the side of the foot or over the top as in diagram opposite.**

# BALANCE

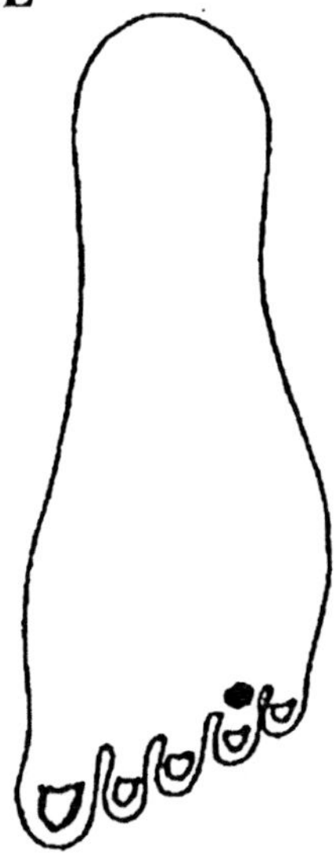

## DIAGRAM 15
## LEFT FOOT
(Top)

## SHOULDER POINT

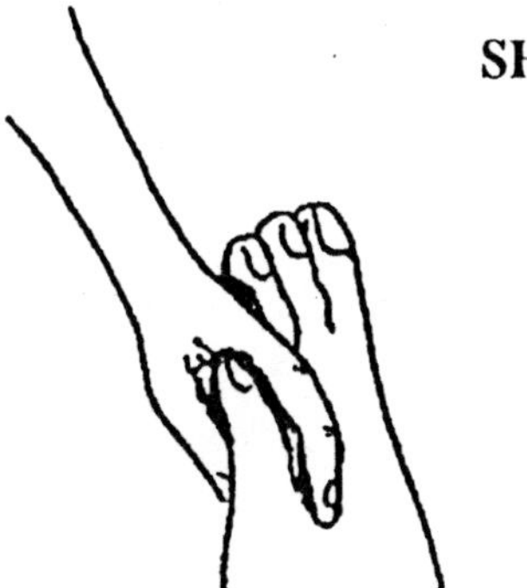

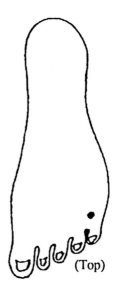

(Outer side)

(Top)

## DIAGRAM 16
## LEFT FOOT

129

## 17.  THYROID / PARATHYROID / THYMUS
(general area treatment)

### Z 1 SOLE

Place the thumb on the diaphragm line at the outer edge of Z 1 toe 1.  Begin
caterpillar like walk towards Z 2 but stop between Z 1 and Z 2.  Turn the
thumb to point towards the toes and work up crease line to between big toe
and toe 2.  Return to start point and repeat entire movement.

## 17A. THYROID

### Z 1 SOLE

Lift the thumb and place it in the centre of the pad of the ball of the foot under
the big toe, move one point up towards the base of the big toe and give three
pressure circles.

## THYROID / PARATHYROID / THYMUS
## (GENERAL AREA TREATMENT)

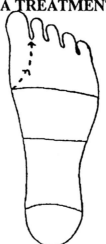

**DIAGRAM 17
LEFT FOOT**
(Sole)

## THYROID

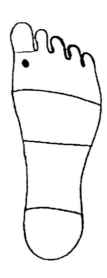

**DIAGRAM 17A
LEFT FOOT**
(Sole)

## 17B.    PARATHYROID

### Z 1 SOLE

Lift the thumb and place it in line with the thyroid on the edge of Z 1 (next to Z 2); move thumb one point up towards the base of the big toe and give three pressure circles.


## 17C.    THYMUS

### Z 1 SOLE

Lift the thumb and place it in line with the thyroid on the ball of the foot on the sole (as close to the edge of the foot as possible while still working on the sole) and give three pressure circles.


## 18.  OESOPHAGUS / TRACHEA

### Z 1 SOLE

Place the thumb on the diaphragm line at the edge of Z 1.  Work from this point up to the base of the big toe.  Return to diaphragm line and continue to work to base of toe until the entire pad has been treated in this way.

**PARATHYROID**

**DIAGRAM 17B
LEFT FOOT**
(Sole)

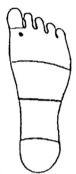

**THYMUS**

**DIAGRAM 17C
LEFT FOOT**
(Sole)

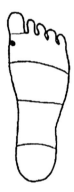

**OESOPHAGUS / TRACHEA**

**DIAGRAM 18
LEFT FOOT**
(Sole)

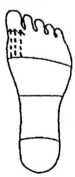

## 19.  CHEST / LUNGS

### Z 2 TO Z 5 SOLE

Put thumb on diaphragm line directly under Z 2.  Work from diaphragm line to base of toes.  Continue to work in this manner until the entire area from Z 2 to Z 5 has been treated.  Repeat movement.

N.B.  This movement can be performed across all four zones.  **It is more usual for the professional therapist to work from the diaphragm towards the toes.**

A note of interest !

When working from diaphragm line Z 5 to base of toe 5 reactions will give indications of shoulder problems.  Treat with pressure circles if necessary.

N.B.  Only the very experienced should treat this area on people with a heart condition.  Medical consent is required.

**DO NOT TREAT IF PACEMAKER FITTED.**

## 20.  CHEST / LUNGS CONTINUED

### Z 1 TO Z 5 TOP OF FOOT

This time work on top of the foot and use the index finger and not the thumb. Start at the base of Z 1, big toe, and work down towards leg to area corresponding to diaphragm line on the sole.  Treat area from Z 1 to Z 5. When area has been treated return to start point and repeat movement.

# CHEST / LUNGS

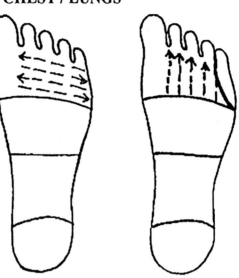

## DIAGRAM 19
## LEFT FOOT
(Sole)

# CHEST / LUNGS - CONTINUED

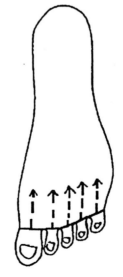

## DIAGRAM 20
## LEFT FOOT
(Top)

# 21. UPPER ABDOMEN

## Z 1 TO Z 5 SOLE

Put thumb on waist line directly under Z 1 on the sole close to the edge of the foot. Work from waist line to diaphragm line. Continue to work in this manner until the entire area between Z 1 and Z 5 has been treated. Return to start point and repeat movement.

N.B. This movement can be performed across all five zones.

**It is more usual for the professional therapist to work across all five zones.**

# 22. CARDIAC / HEART AREA (LEFT FOOT ONLY)

## CHEST AREA

Put the thumb on the diaphragm line on Z 4 pointing towards the toes; press and release X 2. Put the index finger of the same hand on the top of the foot on Z 4 in area corresponding to thumb position on the sole. Work seven gentle massage pressure circles with the index finger. These pressure circles cover the area between Z 4 and Z 2. Keep the thumb in place and remove the index finger. Use the thumb to give seven gentle massage circles on the sole of the foot. As with the index fingers these pressure circles should cover area from Z 4 to Z 2.

**Important!** Do not return to the cardiac area even if sensitivity is felt.

## UPPER ABDOMEN

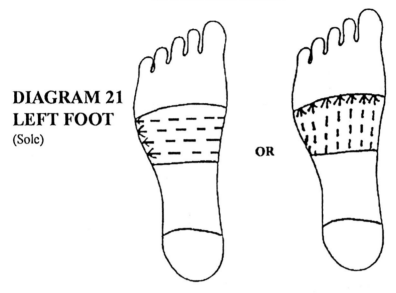

**DIAGRAM 21
LEFT FOOT**
(Sole)

OR

## CARDIAC / HEART AREA

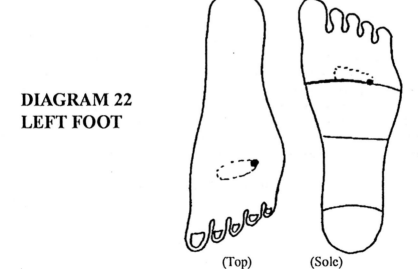

**DIAGRAM 22
LEFT FOOT**

(Top)      (Sole)

## 23.  SPLEEN (LEFT FOOT ONLY)

### Z 3 TO  Z 5 SOLE

Place the thumb facing towards Z 5 one point below the diaphragm line
on Z 3. Work across Z 3 and Z 5 in three straight but overlapping rows. On
completion repeat this movement working this time from Z 5 to Z 3. (Change
hands if necessary ).

N.B. If a reaction occurs during the thumb walk, on completion , the thumb
should be placed between Z 2/4  pointing towards the toes. Press and release
X 3.


## 24.  STOMACH / PANCREAS / DUODENUM

### Z 1 TO Z 3 SOLE

Place thumb one point below diaphragm line on sole (close to edge of foot).
Work from Z 1 to Z 3 across foot in three straight but overlapping rows. On
completion repeat this movement working this time from Z 3 to Z 1 (change
hands if necessary). While most of this area is taken up with the stomach we
are also treating the duodenum/pancreas. The student of anatomy and
physiology will know the area of these structures in the body. **It is necessary
to exercise extreme care when dealing with a diabetic, only a gentle
massage should be given by all but the very well qualified specialist/
therapist.**

**N.B. Stomach ulcers - treat with care. Very light massage over area. No
pressure, as this might cause the ulcer to rupture (consult Doctor)**

**SPLEEN**

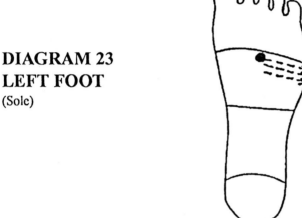

**DIAGRAM 23**
**LEFT FOOT**
(Sole)

**STOMACH / PANCREAS / DUODENUM**

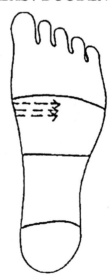

**DIAGRAM 24**
**LEFT FOOT**
(Sole)

# 25. LOWER ABDOMEN / PELVIS / SMALL INTESTINE

## Z 1 TO Z 5 SOLE

Put thumb on heel pad, just below soft flesh. Work with caterpillar like movements from Z 1 to Z 5 - cover area between heel pad and waist line. When area has been treated return to start point and repeat movement. This movement can be performed across all five zones. First working in one direction then the other. **Most professionals favour cross working for this area.**

# 26. SCIATIC LINE

## UP BACK OF LEG

Put one hand under leg, palm uppermost (against leg). Then with a slow, sliding, push movement work from ankle up to behind the knee; return to the start point and repeat X 2. Return to start point again, this time close heel of hand onto leg in a squeezing movement, work up leg to behind knee. Return to start point and repeat X 2.

# LOWER ABDOMEN / PELVIS / SMALL INTESTINE

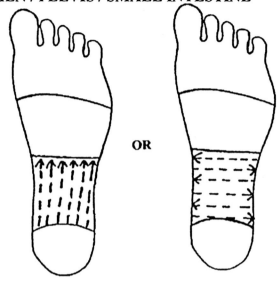

OR

## SCIATIC LINE

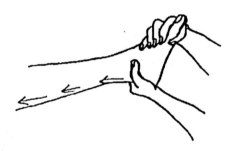

## 27.  SCIATIC LINE - CONTINUED
### BEHIND ANKLE - ACROSS SOLE

Put thumb of one hand (pointing down towards the sole) on the soft flesh area
behind the ankle bone at its highest point.  Work with caterpillar like
movements down behind ankle bone then across the hard heel pad on the sole
of the foot (change hands if necessary) and continue to work with this
movement up behind the other ankle bone to its highest point.  Return to start
point and repeat movement X 2.  ( Total of three ).

## 28.  SPINE
### INNER EDGE OF FOOT

Use the thumb to work with caterpillar like movements down inner edge of
foot from just below nail area on big toe to the  heel.  Follow the curve of the
foot (feeling for the bone).  Repeat movement in opposite direction from heel
to toe, then repeat entire movement.
N.B.  Due to the huge supply of nerves directly from the spinal cord to the
organs of the body, treating the spine works not only on the skeletal and
muscular structure of the area but gives a general treatment to the other organs
of the body.

# SCIATIC LINE - CONTINUED

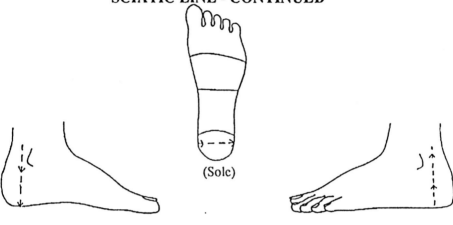

(Sole)

## DIAGRAM 27
## LEFT FOOT

## SPINE

**DIAGRAM 28**
**LEFT FOOT**
(Sole & Medial View)

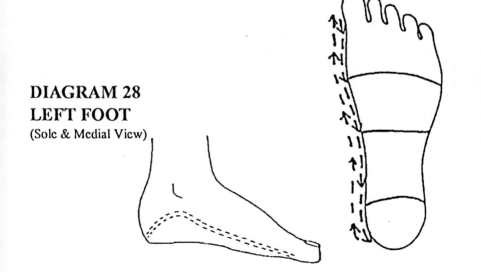

# 29.  SHOULDER / ELBOW / HIP/ KNEE / LOWER BACK

## OUTER EDGE OF FOOT

Use the thumb to work with caterpillar like movement down outer edge of the foot from below nail area on little toe to the heel.  Repeat movement in opposite direction then repeat the entire movement.

# 30.  RECTUM / ANUS / LOWER PELVIC POINT

## Z 1 TO Z 5

Put thumb on outer edge of heel in line with ankle; work with caterpillar movement around behind heel to inside corresponding area; work in a horse shoe shape (change hands if necessary).  Return to start point and repeat movement.

## SHOULDER / ELBOW / HIP /KNEE / LOWER BACK

**DIAGRAM 29
LEFT FOOT**
(Sole)

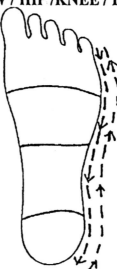

## RECTUM / ANUS / LOWER PELVIC POINT

**DIAGRAM 30
LEFT FOOT**
(Sole)

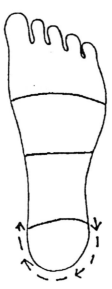

# 31.  KIDNEY / URETER TUBES

## Z 2/3

Place thumb on the waist line between Z 2 and Z 3.  Use left hand.  With tip of thumb pointing towards toes press and release X 2.  Remove thumb, replace thumb and press and release X 2 again.  Swivel thumb around so that tip points towards heel, work down Z 2 to hard heel pad.  Twist hand around, still using thumb, walk up side of foot to centre of the bladder.  Press into centre X 2.

# 32.  BLADDER

## INNER SIDE OF FOOT

The bladder is usually visible as a slightly puffy area.  Place the thumb in the centre of the bladder area then work in points radiating outwards. (Use small caterpillar like movements).
**Do not work back up ureter tubes towards kidney as this may transfer any infection present in the bladder to the kidney.**

| | |
|---|---|
| Line 1 | Work towards Z 2 toe 2 in three points |
| Line 2 | Work towards Z 4 toe 4 in three points |
| Line 3 | Work towards Z 5 toe 5 in three points |
| Line 4 | Work just below line covered by line 3 in same direction but closer to heel pad |

# KIDNEY / URETER TUBES

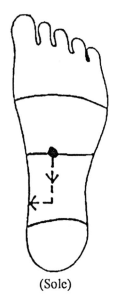

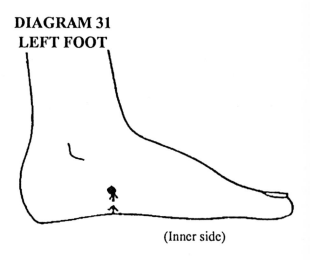

### DIAGRAM 31
### LEFT FOOT

(Sole)

(Inner side)

## BLADDER

## DIAGRAM 32
## LEFT FOOT
(Sole)

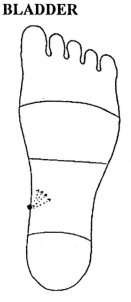

# 33. ADRENALS

Put one thumb on the kidney point pointing towards toes and bring second thumb to meet it on the big toe side. This thumb should be pointing towards the heel. Now both thumbs should be pointing in opposite directions with nails almost parallel. Remove the thumb from the kidney point. With the remaining thumb on the adrenal gland press and release gently X 3.

# 34. UTERUS / PROSTATE

## BELOW INNER ANKLE

Place index finger on inner ankle bone.
Place third finger on tip of heel.
Bend second finger slightly, it will fall in line with the other fingers. When the point of importance has been located by middle finger, remove all three fingers and place the thumb on point where the middle finger rested. Press and release X 3.
This movement can be performed with the index finger on the heel and the third finger on the ankle bone, if this is found to be a more comfortable position for the therapist.
N.B. If IUD is fitted massage with great care. If any previous problems have been experienced then this area should not be treated.

**ADRENALS**

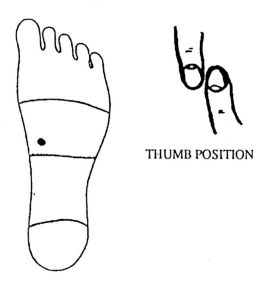

# DIAGRAM 33
# LEFT FOOT
(Sole)

THUMB POSITION

**UTERUS / PROSTATE**

# DIAGRAM 34
# LEFT FOOT
(Inner side)

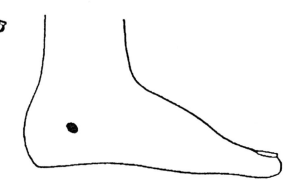

149

## 35.  OVARIES / TESTES

### BELOW OUTER ANKLE

Place index finger on outer ankle bone.
Place third finger on tip of heel.
Bend second finger slightly, it will fall in line with the other fingers. When the point of importance has been located by middle finger, remove all three fingers and place the thumb on point where the middle finger rested. Press and release X 3.
This movement can be performed with the index finger on the heel and the third finger on the ankle bone, if this is found to be a more comfortable position for the therapist.
N.B.  If the client suffers from Acne type skin conditions repeat the pressure X 3.


## 36.  FALLOPIAN TUBES / VAS-DEFERENCE

### TOP OF FOOT

Work with caterpillar like movement from ankle to ankle across crease line between foot and leg.  Repeat this movement in opposite direction.  Then perform the complete movement once more.

# OVARIES / TESTES

**DIAGRAM 35**
**LEFT FOOT**
(Outer side)

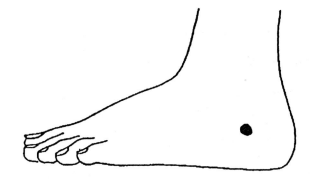

# FALLOPIAN TUBES / VAS-DEFERENCE

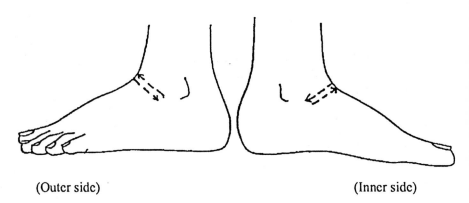

(Outer side)                    (Inner side)

**DIAGRAM 36**
**LEFT FOOT**

# 37. LYMPHATIC / INGUINALS / PELVIC AREA

Place the thumb on the outer edge of the heel (see diagram) pointing upwards towards the leg.
Work up behind the ankle to an area one point higher than the ankle bone, press and release X 2. Turn the thumb around so that tip is pointing towards heel, then slide the thumb back to bottom of the ankle bone. Work around the base of the bone and up in front of the ankle bone to one point higher than the bone. Press and release X 2 (horse shoe shape). Slide the thumb back to the base of the ankle bone. Next work across the leg-foot crease line to the inner ankle. **Change hands** and repeat this entire movement on the other side. Commence at the beginning again and treat the areas of both ankles including the line across the foot.

# 38. BREAST AREA
## Z 2 TO Z 5 TOP OF FOOT

Use pad of index finger to work on the top of the foot in gentle, slow, slide, press and release movement from the base of the toes to an area corresponding to the diaphragm line on the sole. Start movement at the base of toe 2. Work down Z 2, work back between Z 2 and Z 3 using a gentle pull and press movement. Work each zone 2 to 5 in this manner.

# LYMPHATICS / INGUINALS / PELVIC AREA

**DIAGRAM 37
LEFT FOOT**
(Outer side)

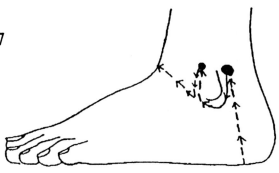

## BREAST AREA

**DIAGRAM 38
LEFT FOOT**
(Top)

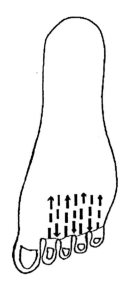

# RETURN TO RIGHT FOOT AND CONTINUE TREATMENT ON BOTH FEET ACCORDING TO ROUTINE (FROM 39 TO 44)

## 39. LYMPHATIC AND GENERAL ABDOMINAL AND CHEST BOOST

### TOP OF BOTH FEET

Use both hands for this movement. Put one hand on each side of the edge of the foot just below the ankle; the fingers should be pointing into the edge of the foot, the thumbs should be on the sole. Slowly move fingers of both hands in a caterpillar like movement towards each other; work up the sides of the foot and on to the top. Treat the area between the ankle and base of toes. This may be repeated once or twice depending on the client's reactions.

## 40. COLON

### SOLES OF BOTH FEET

Put both feet together. Start to work on right foot. Put the thumb pointing towards the toes between Z 4/5 on the hard heel pad just where it meets the soft flesh of the foot. Press firmly. Work the thumb up between Z 4/5 towards the toes to the hepatic flexure (liver area) one point above waist line. Turn the thumb to point towards Z 1 and work across the foot in this direction. At the edge of the foot (Z 1) change to the left foot and work as on the right foot towards Z 5. Stop between Z 4 and Z 5 (splenic flexure ) and turn the thumb to point towards the heel . Work down the foot between Z 4 and Z 5 to the sigmoid flexure at the hard heel pad. Turn the thumb to point towards Z 1; work across Z 4 to Z 1. Turn thumb towards hard heel pad and work down to rectum/anus area. (Repeat entire movement twice).

# LYMPHATIC AND GENERAL ABDOMINAL AND GENERAL CHEST BOOST

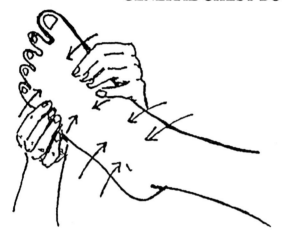

**DIAGRAM 39
BOTH FEET**
(Top)

**COLON**

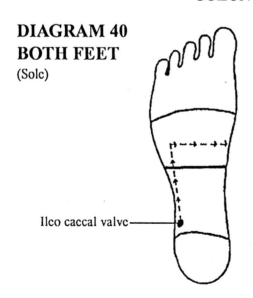

**DIAGRAM 40
BOTH FEET**
(Solc)

Ilco caccal valve

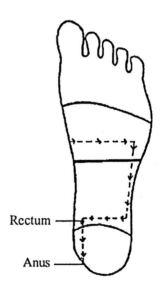

Rectum

Anus

**41.**   RETURN TO TREAT ANY AREAS THAT NEED FURTHER TREATMENT.  (BOTH FEET).

**42.**   WORK ACROSS DIAPHRAGM / SOLAR PLEXUS LINE. TREAT SOLAR PLEXUS.  (BOTH FEET).  START WITH RIGHT FOOT.

**43.**   MASSAGE BOTH FEET STARTING ON RIGHT FOOT.

**44.**   PLACE YOUR THUMBS ON SOLAR PLEXUS POINT OF BOTH FEET AND PRESS GENTLY THREE TIMES.

**45.**   LEAVE CLIENT ON COUCH OR CHAIR ASKING THEM TO RELAX AND NOT TO MOVE .

**46.**   WHILE THE CLIENT IS RELAXING GO AND WASH YOUR HANDS.

**47.**   HELP THE CLIENT OFF THE COUCH /CHAIR AND ASSIST THEM IN DRESSING.

**48.**   MAKE A FURTHER APPOINTMENT IF NECESSARY.

**49.**   COMPLETE CONSULTATION/RECORD CARD.

**50.**   WASH YOU HANDS.

IT SHOULD BE NOTED THAT SOME THERAPISTS LIKE THEIR CLIENTS TO BREATH 'IN' AS THEY PRESS ON THE SOLAR PLEXUS AND 'OUT' AS THEY RELEASE THE PRESSURE.

# SOLAR PLEXUS

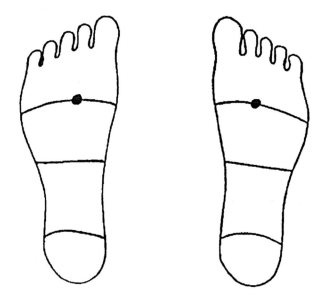

## DIAGRAM 42
## BOTH FEET

# GENERAL OBSERVATIONS OF SPECIFIC REACTIONS

The following list is not meant to be diagnostic in any way. Neither is it intended to be used as a specific treatment routine. However, I believe it is worthy of inclusion in my book, as it has been compiled from my own observations and faithful record keeping throughout my years of treating clients. In Reflexology, as in all other therapies, self education and re-education is very important. These findings might well encourage some therapists to compile and compare data for exchange, study and advancement of Reflexology.

# ACNE

The Pituitary
Thyroid / Parathyroid
The Liver
The Adrenals
The Kidneys
The Ovaries in the Female / Testes, Prostate in the Male
The Lymphatic System

# ALLERGIES

The Adrenals
The Ovaries and Uterus in Female / Testes, Prostate in Males
The Eyes
The Throat / Neck
The Liver
The Lymphatics
The Large and Small Intestines
The Solar Plexus
The Spleen

# ANAEMIA

The Spleen
The Liver

# ANKLES

The Heart
The Kidneys
The Sciatic
The Lymphatics
The Adrenals

# ARMPITS

Advise clients to have any abnormalities in this area checked by their medical practitioner.

The Shoulder
The Lymphatic System, Neck, Underarm and Groin
The Solar Plexus

# ARTHRITIS

The Solar Plexus
The Thyroid and Parathyroid
The Adrenals
The Kidneys
The Arm and Shoulder
The Spine
The Hip, Leg and Knee
The Head and Neck
The Lymphatic System

# ASTHMA

The Solar Plexus
The Pituitary Gland
The Lungs
The Adrenals
The Large and Small Intestines
The Lymphatics
The Thyroid
The Spleen

# BACK ACHE

The Solar Plexus
The Spine
The Shoulder, Arm, Hip and Leg

The Lymphatics
The Kidneys

# BLADDER DISORDERS

The Solar Plexus
The Spleen
The Liver
The Adrenals
The Kidneys
The Bladder
The Lymphatics

# BLOOD PRESSURE

The Solar Plexus
The Pituitary
The Thyroid and Parathyroid
The Heart
The Adrenals
The Kidneys

# BREASTS

Provided a medical opinion has already been sought or the person is advised
to see a medically qualified person, there is no reason why a complete
Reflexology treatment cannot be given.

While we are aware that most breast abnormalities are harmless or if found
not to be so, can be dealt with effectively if caught in time, the Reflexologist
is not in a position to diagnose. He or she would be expected to behave in an
ethical and professional manner in urging the sufferer to consult their Doctor.

# BREAST PROBLEMS BEFORE MENSTRUATION

The Pituitary
The Adrenals
The Kidneys
The Ovaries
The Lymphatics
The Breast
The Solar Plexus

## BRONCHITIS

The Solar Plexus
The Lungs
The Adrenals
The Lymphatics

## BURSITIS

The Adrenals
The Kidneys
The Shoulder
The Arm
The Hip
The Leg
The Lymphatics
The Bladder

# CHOLESTEROL

The Thyroid
The Stomach
The Gall Bladder
The Liver
The Solar Plexus

# COLD

It would be advisable for the therapist to wear a mask when treating this
client.

# COLITIS

The Adrenals
The Large and Small Intestines
The Lymphatic System
The Solar Plexus

# CONSTIPATION

The Solar Plexus
The Stomach
The Pancreas
The Liver
The Gall Bladder
The Adrenals
The Large and Small Intestines
The Lymphatics

# CRAMP (LEG)

The Thyroid and Parathyroid
The Hip, Thigh and Leg
The Sciatic Nerve
The Spine
The Lymphatics
The Solar Plexus

# DIGESTION

The Liver
The Stomach
The Colon
The Solar Plexus
The Head
The Oesophagus
The Lymphatics

# EAR DISORDERS

The Sinuses
The Ear. Eye and Balance Point
The Shoulder
The Spleen
The Solar Plexus

# EYE DISORDERS

The Eye Reflexes
The Cervical Area on Spine
The Shoulder
The Sinuses
The Ears
The Solar Plexus

# FEMALE DISORDER (RELATED TO REPRODUCTIVE SYSTEM)

The Solar Plexus
The Spleen
The Liver
The Kidneys
The Ovaries
The Lymphatics
The Uterus
The Fallopian Tubes

# FLATULENCE (WIND)

The Stomach
The Liver
The Gall Bladder
The Large and Small Intestines
The Ileo Caecal Valve
The Sigmoid Flexure and Descending Colon
The Lymphatics
The Solar Plexus

# FORGETFULNESS (STRESS RELATED)

The Solar Plexus
The Pituitary
The Brain
The Thyroid, Parathyroid and Thymus
The Adrenals
The Pancreas
The Spine
The Shoulder

# GALL BLADDER

The Liver
The Gall Bladder
The Small and Large Intestines
The Kidneys
The Parathyroids
The Lymphatics
The Solar Plexus

# GOUT

The Pituitary
The Spleen
The Adrenals
The Kidneys
The Intestines
The Solar Plexus
The Lymphatics

# HAY FEVER

The Solar Plexus
The Pituitary
The Lungs
The Adrenals
The Spleen

# HEADACHE

The Solar Plexus
The Brain
The Sinuses
The Ear
The Eye
The Pancreas
The Spine
The Shoulder

# HEART DISORDERS

All heart conditions should be checked by a medically qualified practitioner.

# INDIGESTION

The Liver
The Gall Bladder
The Stomach
The Solar Plexus
The Small Intestine
The Large Intestine (colon)

# INFERTILITY (IN FEMALES)

The Solar Plexus
The Pituitary
The Thyroid
The Adrenals
The Ovaries
The Uterus
The Fallopian Tubes

# IMPOTENCE AND INFERTILITY (IN MALES)

The Solar Plexus
The Pituitary
The Brain
The Thyroid and Parathyroid
The Testicles
The Prostate
The Spleen
The Lymphatics

# INSOMNIA

The Solar Plexus
The Brain
The Thyroid and Parathyroid
The Spine
The Shoulder
The Kidneys
The Bladder
The Lymphatics

# KIDNEY DISORDERS

All kidney disorders should be diagnosed by a medically quallified practioner.

The Pituitary
The Thyroid and Parathyroid
The Spleen
The Adrenals
The Kidneys and Ureter
The Bladder and Urethra
The Lymphatics

# LIVER DISORDERS

All liver disorders should be diagnosed by a medicall qualified practioner.

The Thyroid and Parathyroid
The Liver
The Gall Bladder
The Spleen
The Kidneys
The Lymphatics

# LUNG DISORDERS

Conditions of the lung, like all major organs, need to be investigated by a medically qualified practioner.

The Solar Plexus and Diaphragm
The Lungs
The Adrenals
The Lymphatics

# MENOPAUSE

The Solar Plexus
The Pituitary
The Thyroid and Parathyroid
The Ovaries
The Uterus
The Brain
The Lymphatics

# MENSTRUAL (PREMENSTRUAL TENSION)

The Pituitary
The Brain
The Thyroid and Parathyroid
The Adrenals
The Kidneys
The Ovaries
The Uterus
The Spine
The Solar Plexus

# MIGRAINE

The Solar Plexus
The Brain
The Pituitary
The Heart
The Adrenals
The Kidneys
The Large and Small Intestines
The Sinuses
The Spine and Shoulder

# NAUSEA

The Solar Plexus
The Brain
The Stomach
The Ear Reflex
The Balance Point
The Intestines (Large and Small)
The Adrenals

# SCIATICA

The Sciatic
The Intestines (Large and Small)
The Spine
The Hip, Thigh and Leg
The Adrenals
The Sciatic Nerve
The Solar Plexus

# SINUSITIS

The Pituitary
The Sinuses
The Intestines (Large and Small)
The Adrenals
The Lymphatic System

# SKIN DISORDERS

The Solar Plexus
The Pituitary
The Thyroid
The Parathyroid
The Thymus
The Adrenals
The Liver
The Kidneys
The Gonads (Ovaries or Testicles)
The Lymphatic System

# STRESS

The Solar Plexus
The Pituitary
The Thyroid and Parathyroid
The  Lungs
The Kidneys
The Spine
The Shoulder, Hip, Leg
The Lymphatics

# ULCERS (DIGESTIVE)

The Solar Plexus
The Stomach
The Intestines (Large and Small)
The Adrenals
The Liver
The Lymphatics

# VARICOSE VEINS

The Heart
The Adrenals
The Hip, Thigh, and Leg
The Solar Plexus
The Intestines (Large and Small)
The Lymphatics

# REVISION QUESTIONS

1     Who brought Reflexology to America?

2     Name the American woman who specialized in Reflexology.

3     How do the reflex points of Reflexology differ from the reflex points of the nervous system?

5     In Reflexology what is meant by reflex points?

6     Where are the Transverse Lines found?

7     What are the Longitudinal Zones?

8     What are the Crystals?

9     There are many reasons why a treatment may not be performed. List not less than twelve.

10    Would you treat an Epileptic?

11    Are there any special precautions when treating a Diabetic?

12    What might happen if you overtreated a client?

13    Is it within the powers of a Reflexologist to refer people to their own Doctor?

14    Give a list of Do Not's in Reflexology.

15    List seven rules of personal hygiene.

16    Name a contagious condition that affects the feet.

17    What should you do with the foot bowl after use?

18    With what should you cover the knee and foot rest?

19    Why is the comfort of both Therapist and Client important?

20    How should the client be kept warm?

21    While performing the initial foot massage what is the Therapist looking for or observing on the feet?

22    Why is it important for the client to see the Therapist's face?

23    Why is it not advisable to use oil, cream or talc in Reflexology?

24    If a Therapist thinks it is necessary to treat with an oil, cream or talc, then at what stage in the treatment can these products be used?

25    What home care advice would you give to a client with excessively sweaty feet?

26    How much time would you allow for a first visit?

27    What sort of situation would dictate that the treatment should be given for 5/10 minutes instead of 40/45?

28    How does treatment of a child differ from treatment of an adult?

29    How often would you give a Reflexology treatment over the space of eight days?

30    What action does the Therapist take when a Crystal or sensitivity is felt?

31    Name the first area to be treated in the Reflexology Routine.

32    In what Zone does the head and brain lie?

33    Where would you massage for the Pituitary?

34    Over what area on the foot is the Spine treated?

35    In the 'Reflexology Routine' what organ would you be working on between Z 1 to Z 5 between waist and pelvic floor line?

36 According to the routine in this book which would you treat first, the Kidney or the Bladder?

37 Define 'Contra Indicated'.

38 What sort of reaction might a client display during treatment?

39 Might a client suffer any reactions between visits to the Therapist and if so what type of reactions might be expected?

40 Why is a Consultation Card necessary?

# SOME COMMON QUESTIONS ANSWERED

Q    Are all Aromatherapists qualified Reflexologists?

A    No. Some Aromatherapists will have undertaken a separate course to qualify them in the field of Reflexology.

Q    I have been told that Reflexology is part of Aromatherapy. Is this true?

A    No! Some Aromatherapists do press on some Reflexology points in order to help them choose an oil for their Aromatherapy treatment; but this cannot be classified as Reflexology. However fortunately this is becoming a practice less often performed by the well qualified Aromatherapist.

Q    Are all Beauty Therapists Reflexologists?

A    No. Beauty Therapists who hold qualifications to undertake face and body treatments will have studied anatomy, physiology and massage. However, this does not qualify them as Reflexologists.

Q    Does the Reflexologist have to be insured?

A    All professional people should be insured.

Q    How can a Therapist get insurance to practise?

A    Therapists gaining their training through a recognised establishment will be given details of professional bodies/societies for membership and insurance.

Q    Where can I get information about courses?

A    By writing to one of the organisations listed on page 203, enclosing a stamped addressed envelope for your reply.

Q    If I experience problems finding local training at times to suit me how do I get help?

A    The author will help where possible in advising on seminars, lectures and open learning facilities run by her own organisation, Renbardou Training, but she is unable to enter into any other correspondence.
(addresses can be found at the back of the book )

# SOME HELPFUL DIAGRAMS

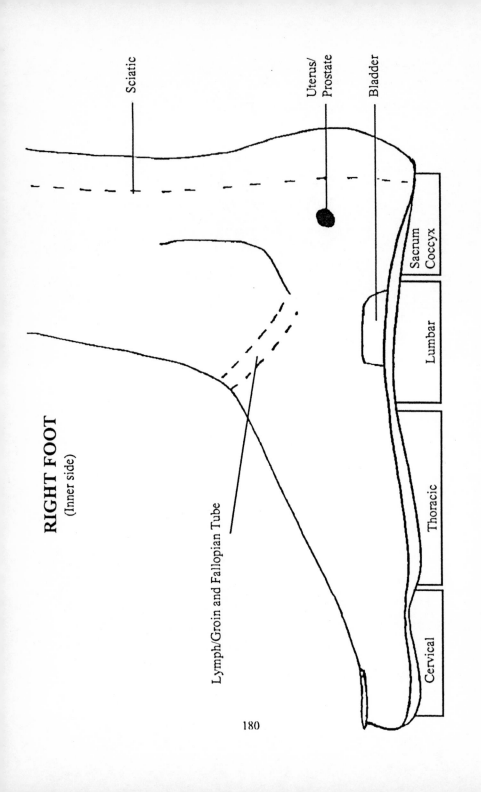

**RIGHT FOOT**
(Inner side)

Sciatic

Uterus/Prostate

Bladder

Sacrum Coccyx

Lumbar

Thoracic

Cervical

Lymph/Groin and Fallopian Tube

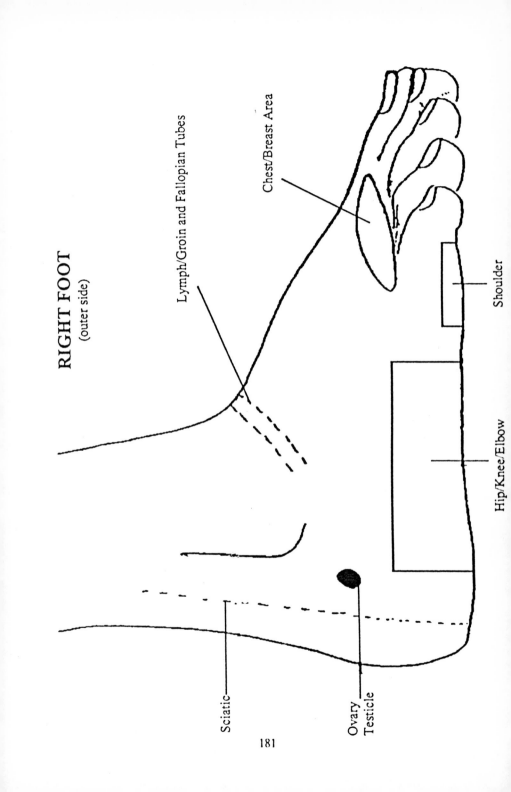

RIGHT FOOT
(outer side)

Lymph/Groin and Fallopian Tubes

Chest/Breast Area

Shoulder

Hip/Knee/Elbow

Sciatic

Ovary
Testicle

181

# RIGHT FOOT
## (Sole)

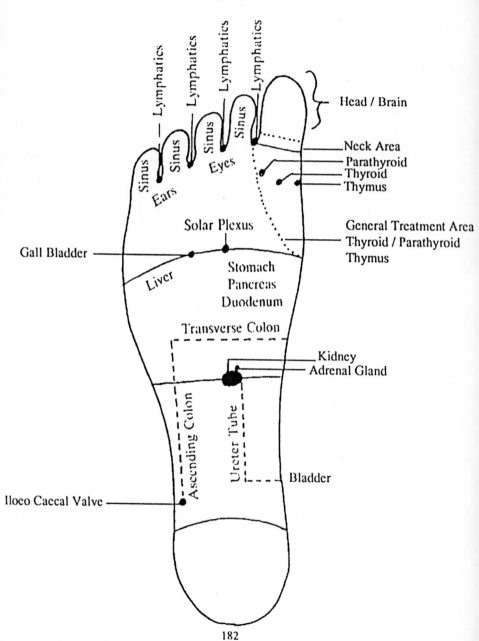

Lymphatics

Sinus

Ears

Eyes

Head / Brain

Neck Area

Parathyroid

Thyroid

Thymus

Solar Plexus

General Treatment Area
Thyroid / Parathyroid
Thymus

Gall Bladder

Liver

Stomach
Pancreas
Duodenum

Transverse Colon

Kidney

Adrenal Gland

Ascending Colon

Ureter Tube

Bladder

Iloeo Caecal Valve

# LEFT FOOT
## (Sole)

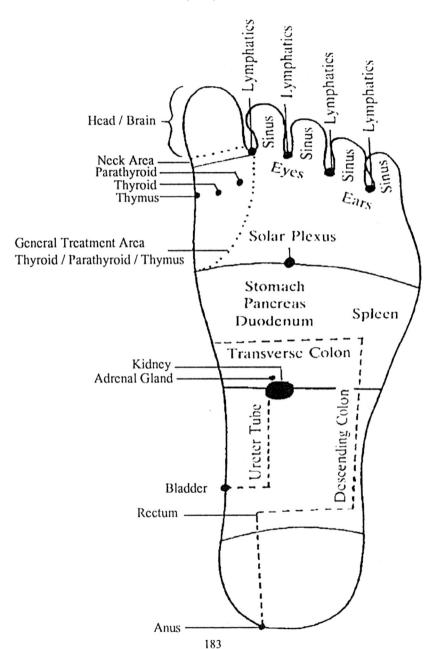

Head / Brain

Neck Area
Parathyroid
Thyroid
Thymus

Lymphatics
Lymphatics
Lymphatics
Lymphatics

Sinus
Sinus
Eyes
Sinus
Sinus
Ears
Sinus

General Treatment Area
Thyroid / Parathyroid / Thymus

Solar Plexus

Stomach
Pancreas
Duodenum

Spleen

Transverse Colon

Kidney
Adrenal Gland

Ureter Tube

Descending Colon

Bladder
Rectum

Anus

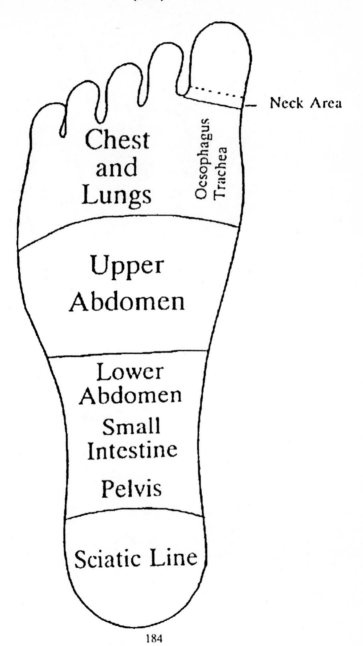

Neck Area

Chest
and
Lungs

Oesophagus
Trachea

Upper
Abdomen

Lower
Abdomen

Small
Intestine

Pelvis

Sciatic Line

# LEFT FOOT
### (Sole)

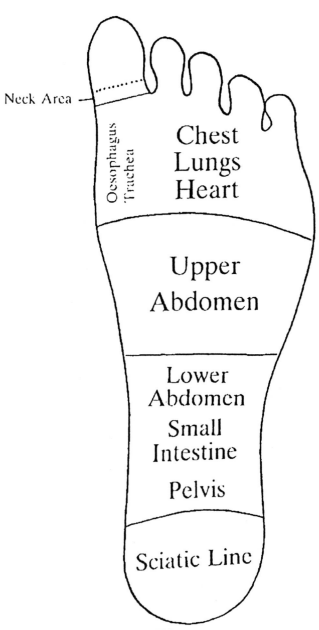

Neck Area —

Oesophagus
Trachea

Chest
Lungs
Heart

Upper
Abdomen

Lower
Abdomen

Small
Intestine

Pelvis

Sciatic Line

# RIGHT FOOT
## (Sole)

Shoulder
Arm
Hip
Leg
Knee
Lower Back

Spine

# ZONES OF THE HAND

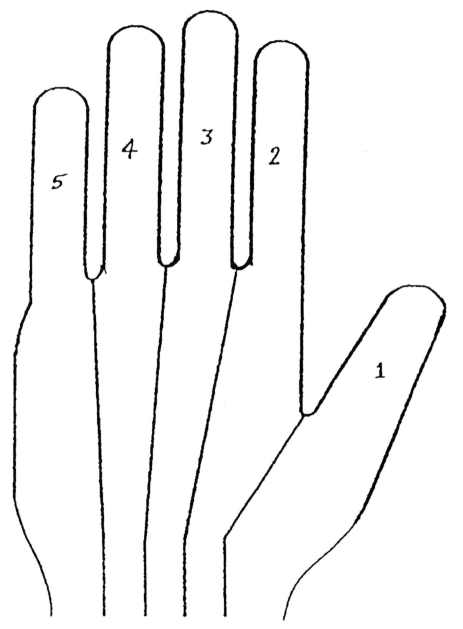

# RIGHT HAND
## (Back)

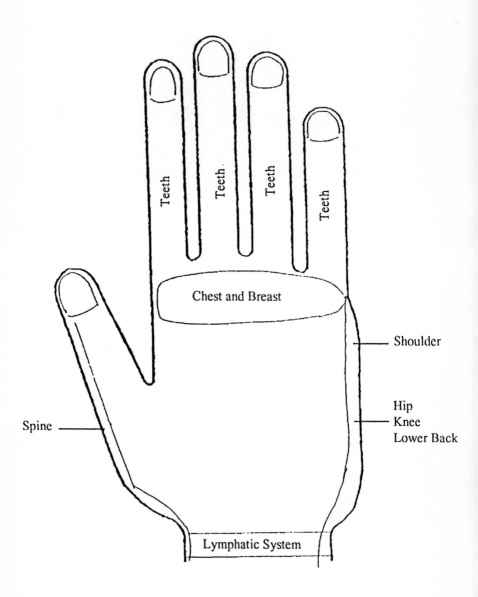

Teeth

Teeth

Teeth

Teeth

Chest and Breast

Shoulder

Hip
Knee
Lower Back

Spine

Lymphatic System

# LEFT HAND
## (Back)

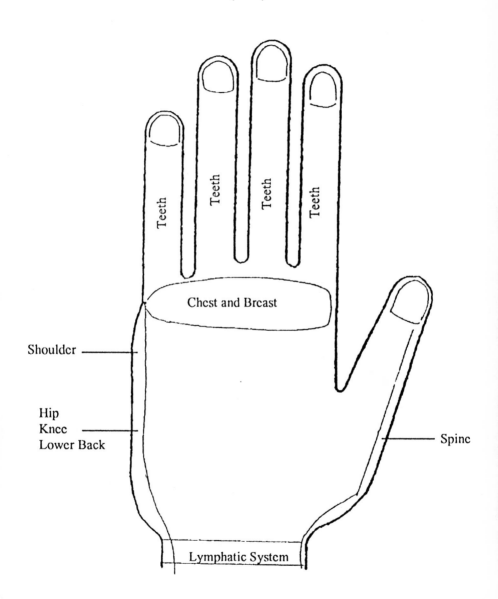

Teeth

Teeth

Teeth

Teeth

Chest and Breast

Shoulder

Hip
Knee
Lower Back

Spine

Lymphatic System

# RIGHT HAND
## (Palm)

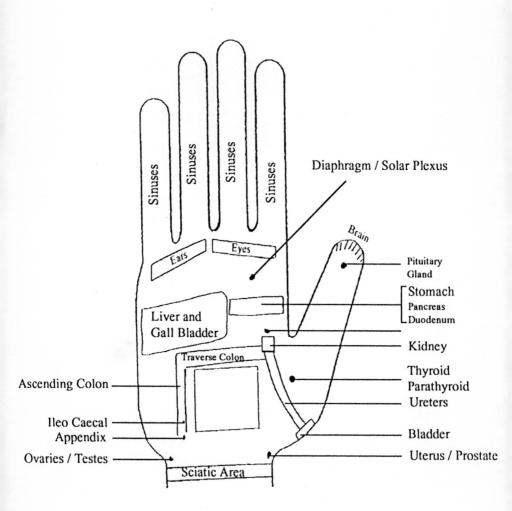

# LEFT HAND
### (Palm)

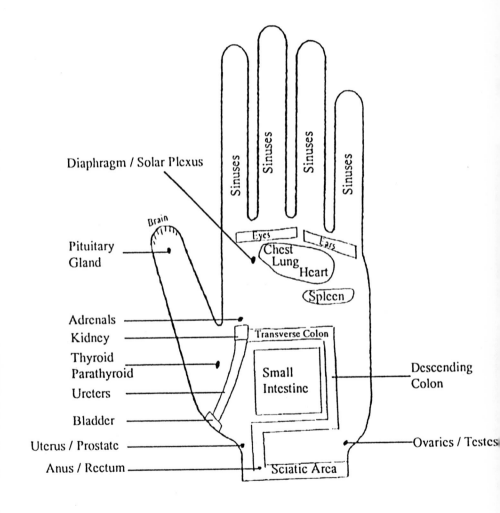

Diaphragm / Solar Plexus

Sinuses

Sinuses

Sinuses

Sinuses

Brain

Eyes

Ears

Chest
Lung
Heart

Spleen

Pituitary
Gland

Adrenals

Kidney

Transverse Colon

Thyroid
Parathyroid

Small
Intestine

Descending
Colon

Ureters

Bladder

Uterus / Prostate

Ovaries / Testes

Anus / Rectum

Sciatic Area

# A HOLDING TECHNIQUE

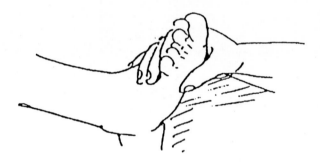

# HOLDING TECHNIQUE WHEN TREATING
## CHEST OR ABDOMEN

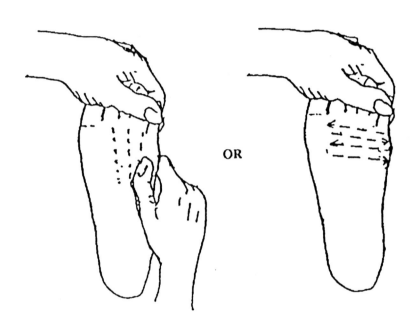

OR

# HOLDING TECHNIQUE WHEN
# TREATING TOP OF FOOT

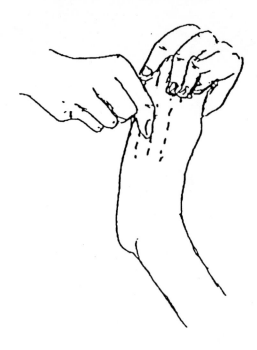

# BENDING BACK THE TOES

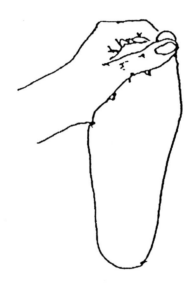

# FOOT SUPPORT / HOLDING TECHNIQUE

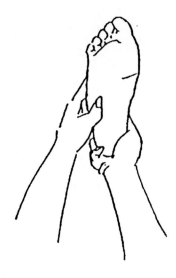

# WORKING ON SOLAR PLEXUS

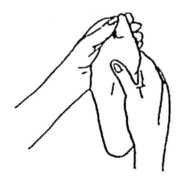

# MEMORY JOGGER

| | |
|---|---|
| 1 | Diaphragm / Solar Plexus |
| 2 | Head / Brain |
| 3 | Front of neck |
| 4 | Back of neck |
| 5 | Occipital |
| 6 | Ear / Mastoid Process |
| 7 | Pituitary |
| 8 | Sinuses |
| 9 | Teeth |
| 10 | Lymphatics of Head and Neck |
| 11 | Ears / Eyes |
| 12 | Eye point |
| 13 | Ear Point |
| 14 | Eustachian Tube |
| 15 | Balance |
| 16 | Shoulder |
| 17 | Thyroid / Parathyroid / Thymus Area |
| 17a | Thyroid |
| 17b | Parathyroid |
| 17c | Thymus |
| 18 | Oesphagus / Trachea |
| 19 | Chest Lungs - Sole of Foot |
| 20 | Chest Lungs - Top of Foot |
| 21 | Upper Abdomen |
| 22 | Right Foot Only - Gall Bladder |
| 23 | Right Foot Only - Liver |
| 24 | Stomach / Pancreas / Duodenum |
| 25 | Lower abdomen / Pelvis / Small Intestine |
| 26 | Sciatic Line |
| 27 | Sciatic Line - continued |
| 28 | Spine |
| 29 | Shoulder / Hip / Knee / Lower Back |
| 30 | Rectum / Anus / Lower Pelvis |
| 31 | Kidney / Ureter Tubes |
| 32 | Bladder |
| 33 | Adrenals |
| 34 | Uterus / Prostate |
| 35 | Ovaries / Testes |
| 36 | Fallopian Tubes / Vas-Deference |
| 37 | Lymphatics / Inguinals / Pelvic Area |
| 38 | Breast Area |
| 40 | Lymphatic / General Abdominal / Chest Boost - Tops Both Feet |
| 41 | Colon - Both Feet |
| 42 | Solar Plexus |
| 43 | Massage - Both Feet |
| 44 | Solar Plexus - Both Feet at the same time. |

## GENERAL NOTES ON BECOMING A QUALIFIED
## REFLEXOLOGIST

As I have said before, it is not easy to learn Reflexology from a book.

For the Therapist who would like to work as a professional I would venture to say it is almost impossible without years of practice, trial and error to achieve the standard of a professional without some help and guidance in the practical and theoretical field.

No book which I have found, or indeed this one which I myself have written, can possibly contain all the information on reflex zones, referral zones, reactions to treatments, anatomy and physiology, disorders and diseases or give reasons why there might be some slight differences in the location of organ /reflex zones.

A course of Reflexology for the professional Therapist will answer all these questions. It will also give the student time for practical and theoretical work whilst under supervision.

All budding Reflexologists with a thirst for knowledge who do not hold a qualification in anatomy and physiology should buy and study a simple text book on the subject ; and it would be even more advantageous if the opportunity presents itself, to attend a part time course ( day or evening ) in Human Biology at your local college/school of Continuing Education and Training. Either or both of these courses of action will make life much easier when and if you decide to become a professional Therapist.

One other book which I feel sure would be invaluable is a good simple to follow Medical Dictionary.

# AND FINALLY....

Practicing Reflexologists should, in my opinion, hold a certificate in First Aid and attend a course on Nutrition.

# STUDENT NOTES

# STUDENT NOTES

## OTHER BOOKS IN THE
## STEP BY STEP SERIES


STEP BY STEP    AROMATHERAPY

By Renée Tanner


STEP BY STEP    BASIC ANATOMY & PHYSIOLOGY
FOR STUDENTS

By Renée Tanner


STEP BY STEP    BASIC MASSAGE

By Renée Tanner

## ADDRESSES OF ORGANISATIONS

(enclose A4 size s.a.e. with Enquiry )

**The International Federation of Reflexologists**
78 Edridge Road
Croydon
Surrey
England
CR0 1EF
Tel : 081 667 9458

**International Examinations Board. (I.E.B.)**
P.O. Box 281
London
WC1B 3NW
Tel : 071 436 3606

# ALTERNATIVE THERAPIES COURSES

**Colette McCabe,**
Rathganny
Multy Farnham,
Co. West Meath,
Ireland.

**Renée Tanner**
Renbardou Beauty and Alternative Therapies Training Centre.
**(All correspondence for both London and Surrey centres**
**should be addressed to :)**
Acorn House,
Cherry Orchard Road,
Croydon, Surrey, England CR0 6BA
Tel : 081 686 4781

Kathy. Gunning.

# STEP BY STEP
# REFLEXOLOGY

**A SIMPLE STEP BY STEP EASY TO FOLLOW GUIDE WHICH EXPLAINS THE PRINCIPLES AND APPLICATIONS OF REFLEXOLOGY OF THE FEET.**

**DOUGLAS BARRY PUBLICATIONS**
**21 LAUD STREET**
**CROYDON, SURREY**
**CR0 1SU**

# ABOUT THE AUTHOR

Renée Tanner is head of training for the Renbardou Group based at their centres in Central London and in Surrey.  With almost 30 years of experience within the profession, she is a lecturer and author of international repute.  Renée is also well respected for her numerous contributions to Radio, Television and Journals
( publications for both the Profession and general public magazines).

# REFLEXOLOGY MASSAGE
# A HANDBOOK FOR EVERYONE

FIRST PUBLISHED IN THE U.K. 1990
STEP BY STEP REFLEXOLOGY
REVISED SECOND EDITION 1991

# COPYRIGHT 1990
# © RENÉE TANNER

All Rights Reserved.No part of this publication/document may be reproduced or transmitted in any form or by any means, electronic or mechanical, including photocopying, recording, or any information storage and retrieval system, without permission in writing from the author, Renée Tanner. Written in 1990.

British Library - A CIP Catalogue
record for this book is available
from the British Library.

I.S.B.N. 0-9516203-1-2
Published in Great Britain by
Douglas Barry Publications,
21 Laud Street,
Croydon, Surrrey.
CR0 1SU.

**DEDICATED TO THE MEMORY
OF MY LATE PARENTS**

# ACKNOWLEDGEMENTS

I am indebted to many people who assisted me in the writing of this book. Firstly I would like to thank my family for all the time, energy and constant encouragement given during the writing of the manuscript.

Also my many Clients, Friends, and Students both past and present who encouraged me to put my ideas down on paper and without whom this book might never have been written.

Finally I wish to place on record my thanks and appreciation for the help support and encouragement given to me by my friend Anneke Van Der Mey.

# CONTENTS